Self-assessment in dermatology

USING CLINICAL CASES

Copyright © 2018 Grupo Asís Biomedia, SL
Plaza Antonio Beltrán Martínez n.º 1, planta 8 - letra I
(Centro empresarial El Trovador)
50002 Zaragoza - Spain

First printing: April 2018

This book was originally published in Spanish under the title:
Autoevaluación en dermatología a través de casos clínicos
© 2017 Grupo Asís Biomedia, SL
ISBN Spanish edition: 978-84-17225-02-5

Translation:
Owen Howard

ISBN: 978-84-17225-58-2
DL: Z 567-2018

Design, layout and printing:
Servet editorial - Grupo Asís Biomedia, SL
www.grupoasis.com
info@grupoasis.com

Servet is the publishing house of Grupo Asís

Warning:

Veterinary science is constantly evolving, as are pharmacology and the other sciences. Inevitably, it is therefore the responsibility of the veterinary surgeon to determine and verify the dosage, the method of administration, the duration of treatment and any possible contraindications to the treatments given to each individual patient, based on his or her professional experience. Neither the publisher nor the author can be held liable for any damage or harm caused to people, animals or properties resulting from the correct or incorrect application of the information contained in this book.

Self-assessment in dermatology

USING CLINICAL CASES

Ana María Ríos Boeta

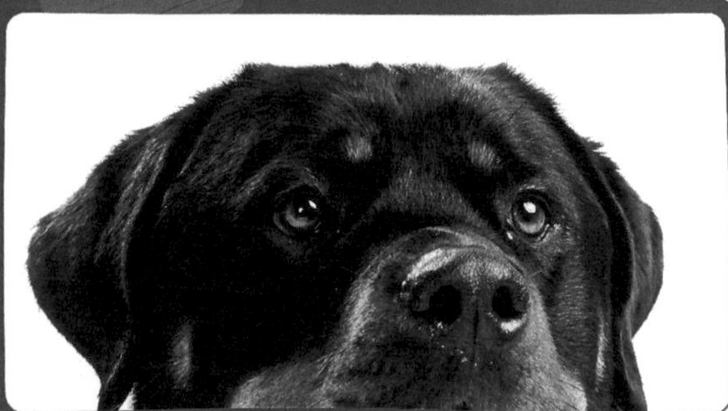

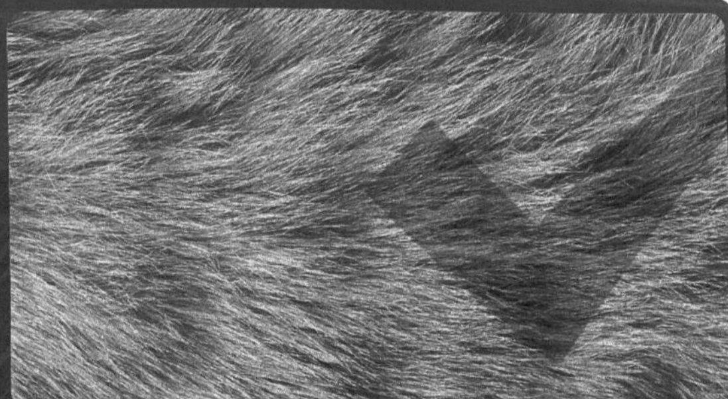

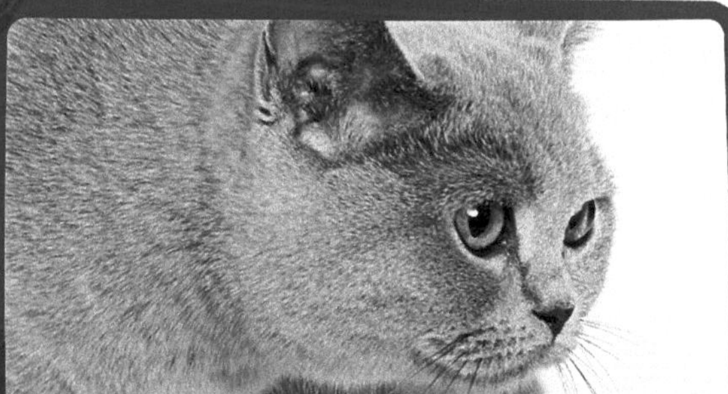

SERVET

This book is dedicated to my children, Marta and Matías,
and all my pets (*Nero*, *Curra*, *Nana,* and *Bochito*).

Acknowledgements

To all my colleagues at the Puchol Veterinary Hospital, and especially its director José Luis Puchol, for giving me the opportunity to work on such an interesting project in such a stimulating environment.

To all the veterinary surgeons and students with whom I have worked at the Delicias Veterinary Medical Centre, the Veterinary Teaching Hospital of Alfonso X University, and the Ciudad de los Ángeles Veterinary Clinic. Without a team effort, this book would never have materialised.

To my colleagues, from all over the world, who specialise in veterinary dermatology; thank you for sharing your knowledge and experience.

And especially to all my patients, big and small, who, together with their owners, teach me a little more each day.

The author

Ana María Ríos Boeta

Degree in veterinary science from the Complutense University of Madrid. PhD in Veterinary Sciences and Master's in Research Methodology in Health Sciences from Alfonso X University. Certified in dermatology by AVEPA (Spanish Small Animal Veterinary Association) and recipient of a master's in dermatology from the ESAVS (European School of Advanced Veterinary Studies).

Currently, she heads the Dermatology Service of the Puchol Veterinary Hospital (Madrid).

Ana María Ríos is a full member of the ESVD (European Society of Veterinary Dermatology), a founding member of GEDA (Specialist Dermatology Group of AVEPA), and has been a board member of AVEPA and President of the GEDA. She is the creator and coordinator of the veterinary dermatology teaching website www.cuestiondpiel.wordpress.com.

Foreword

Dermatological conditions, particularly those affecting small animals, account for a significant proportion of consultations in veterinary practice. Indeed, veterinary surgeons attend to patients with skin conditions on an almost daily basis.

The knowledge needed to perform effectively in clinical practice is acquired through study, always applying a rigorous method. If we have acquired knowledge, but are unable to both understand and apply it, then we have not yet acquired wisdom. In this book, the author shares her knowledge and wisdom in the field of dermatology in the form of a self-assessment book, in which the reader is provided with a series of clinical cases, each with a set of corresponding questions and answers. Using a methodical and educational approach, the book describes the clinical presentation, differential diagnosis, diagnostic tests, and relevant treatments corresponding to the most common dermatological processes and diseases.

The author of this book is a veterinary surgeon of recognised prestige, with extensive clinical experience. As a clinical veterinary surgeon, I would like to thank Ana Ríos for her excellent work, and above all I wish to highlight her enthusiasm and scientific rigour, without which the final result would not have been of such extraordinary quality. I have no doubt that this book will be of great help to clinical veterinary surgeons who wish to test their knowledge and improve their ability to deal with the daily challenges presented by dermatology cases. Enjoy!

Artur Font
Ldo Vet. AVEPA-certified (Internal Medicine)
ECVIM-CA Diplomate (Internal Medicine)
Ars Veterinary Hospital

Preface

This book provides a general review of veterinary dermatology using a non-traditional approach, allowing the reader to assess their own knowledge of the clinical cases presented. For me, daily practice represents both a constant challenge and a source of continuous learning. Thanks to my love of photography and my passion for microscopy, I have collected a wealth of information on individual clinical cases that I have always wished to share with colleagues interested in this particular veterinary specialty.

The book focuses on the diagnosis of skin diseases, an intellectual exercise that clinicians must constantly perform, and requires the reader to select the most appropriate diagnostic procedures. The case studies presented include horses, goats, and other species with which I am lucky enough to work with occasionally. Regardless of the species in question, the scientific protocol is always the same. In an attempt to replicate the reality of clinical practice, this book does not include an index, for when a patient enters our practice we cannot know a priori whether their condition corresponds to, for example, an allergic, infectious, or neoplastic process. I have made a particular effort to make the content as varied, current, and enjoyable as possible, and I hope you enjoy reading it as much as I enjoyed writing it.

Ana María Ríos

More clinical cases are available in the digital version.

Case 1

Case presentation

An intact male Maltese, aged 9 years, weighing 5.4 kg, was brought to the clinic by his owners for assessment of pruritus. He had started chewing at his legs, and was diagnosed by his usual veterinary surgeon with flea-bite allergic dermatitis. Treatment with prednisone, itraconazole, amoxicillin/clavulanic acid, and a hydrolysed diet resulted in no improvement. At the time when he was taken to the clinic, the patient was not receiving any medication. He had generalised pruritus, and his owners reported that he appeared dejected and had lost weight. He did not live with other animals and had not received any external antiparasitic treatment during the preceding year. The owners themselves had no lesions. The patient's body condition was poor, and the dermatological examination revealed lesions on the face and on the skin of the abdomen and trunk (Figs. 1.1 and 1.2).

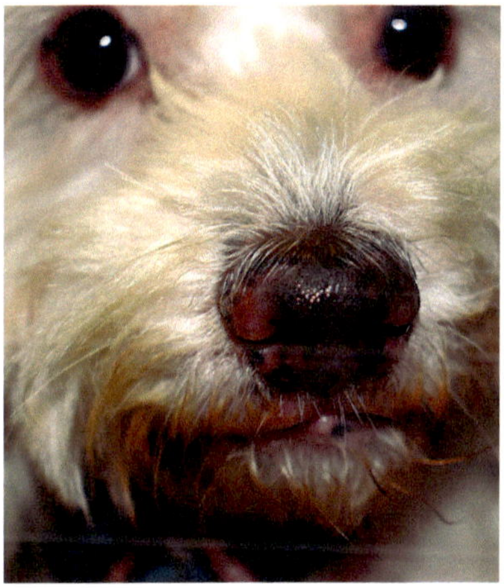

Figure 1.1. Lesions on the patient's face.

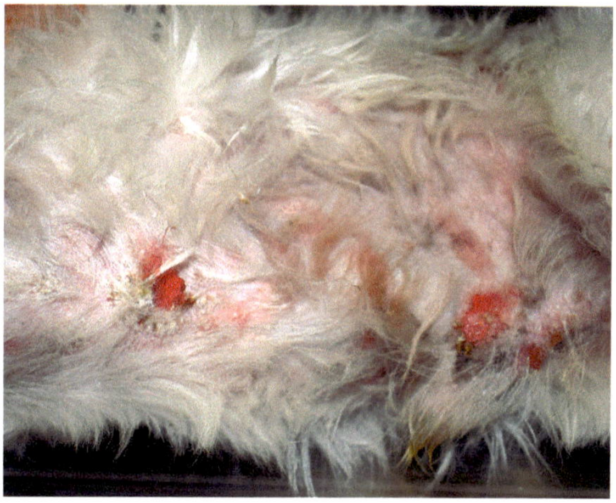

Figure 1.2. Lesions on the abdomen.

Questions

1. What skin lesions do you see in this patient?
2. What are the most likely diagnoses?
3. What diagnostic tests would you perform?
4. What are the treatment options?

Answers Case 1

1 What skin lesions do you see in this patient?

This dog exhibits alopecia and erythema on the eyelids and lips, depigmentation of the muzzle with erosive and crusted lesions, and loss of the normal anatomy of the muzzle. In addition, ulcerative and crusted lesions and scaling are evident on the skin of the abdomen.

2 What are the most likely diagnoses?

The patient's weight loss suggests a chronic and systemic process. Lesions on the muzzle with depigmentation and erosive and crusted lesions suggest an inflammatory process, which could be due to a variety of causes:

- Autoimmune diseases, such as pemphigus foliaceus or discoid or systemic lupus.
- Infections, such as leishmaniasis and superficial or deep mycoses.
- Environmental causes, e.g. solar dermatitis.
- Tumours, e.g. epitheliotropic lymphoma.

The generalised ulcerative lesions and the animal's condition suggest a serious systemic disease such as epitheliotropic lymphoma, leishmaniasis, a severe immune-mediated process, a drug reaction, or vasculitis.

3 What diagnostic tests would you perform?

Lesion cytology: this is a simple, rapid, and inexpensive test that can be highly informative. Lesion cytology indicated a predominance of round lymphoblast-like cells (Figs. 1.3 and 1.4). This profile is compatible with epitheliotropic lymphoma. A biopsy was performed to confirm the diagnosis.

4 What are the treatment options?

Epitheliotropic lymphoma is one of the forms of lymphoma that affects canine species. It is usually caused by T cells and responds poorly to chemotherapy. The current recommended treatment is a combination of prednisone and lomustine.

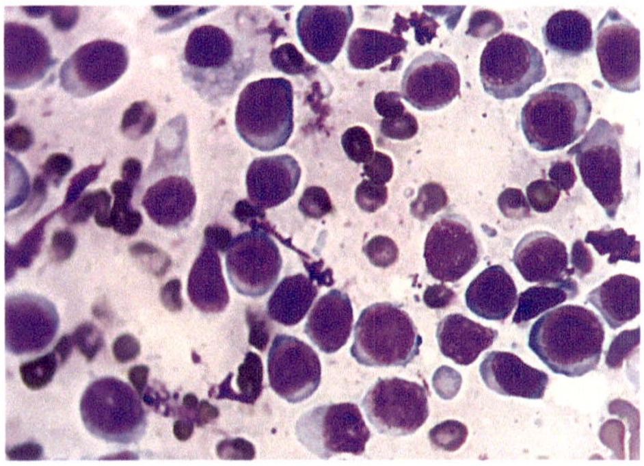

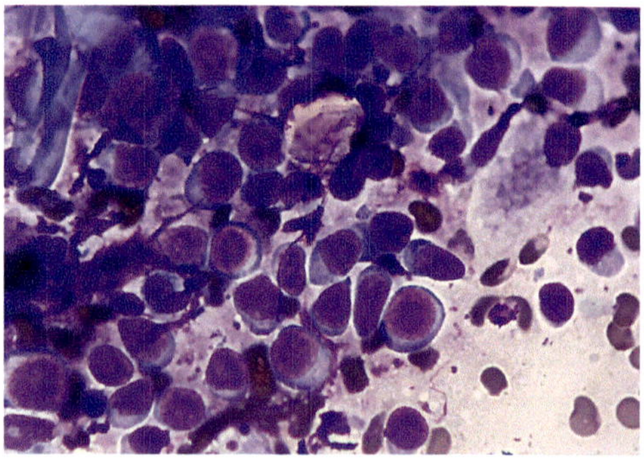

Figures 1.3 and 1.4. Cytology of the lesions.

Case 2

Case presentation

A 7-year-old, spayed female Yorkshire Terrier was brought to the clinic with poor haircoat condition, pruritus, and a foul body odour, signs that had first appeared 2 years earlier. She had been spayed for treatment of a pyometra, after which the foul odour had developed. By the time she was taken to the clinic she had developed marked pruritus and alopecia. Treatment with fatty acids and shampoos (for sensitive skin) every 15 days had resulted in no improvement. Her general condition was good, and her water consumption was normal. Her diet consisted of dry food for small breeds. She lived with other dogs and cats that were healthy, and her owners had no lesions. She had received treatment for the control of internal, but not external, parasites. She lived in an apartment with a patio and garden and had not left the city during the previous 6 months. The general examination revealed no findings of note, except for the presence of periodontal disease and bilateral patellar dislocation.

In the dermatological examination, poor haircoat condition and a foul body odour were evident (Fig. 2.1), as well as generalised oily seborrhoea with multifocal alopecia and erythema, crusts, hyperpigmented plaques, and scaling on the trunk and ventral aspect of the neck (Figs. 2.2 and 2.3). Seborrhoeic otitis was evident in both ears, and the patient had seborrhoeic dermatitis.

Questions

1. What could be complicating this seborrhoeic condition and causing the foul odour and pruritus?
2. What diagnostic tests would you perform to confirm this?
3. What are the most common causes of oily seborrhoea in dogs?

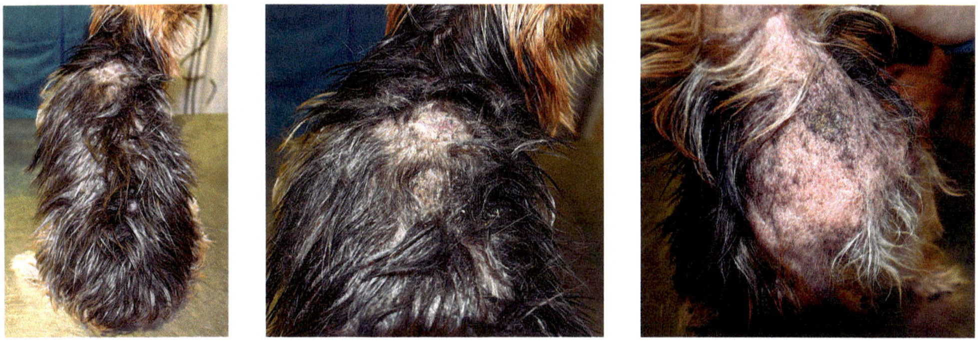

Figures 2.1–2.3. Appearance of the patient's lesions.

Answers Case 2

1 What could be complicating this seborrhoeic condition and causing the foul odour and pruritus?

The most common causes of pruritus and foul odour in seborrhoeic dermatitis are secondary infections, although the odour could be caused exclusively by seborrhoea.

2 What diagnostic tests would you perform to confirm this?

Cytology can help in the diagnosis of secondary infections. In this patient, surface cytology revealed a population of cells consisting mainly of corneocytes and occasional neutrophils. A large number of extracellular coccoid bacteria and yeasts of the species *Malassezia pachydermatis* were evident (Figs. 2.4 and 2.5). This profile is compatible with overgrowth of bacteria and *Malassezia.*

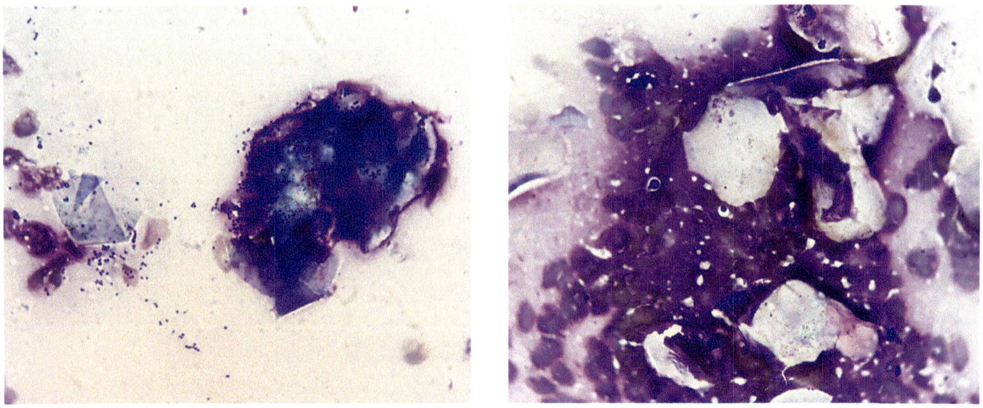

Figures 2.4 and 2.5. Cytological images in which numerous bacteria and yeasts are observed.

3 What are the most common causes of oily seborrhoea in dogs?

The most common causes of seborrhoeic dermatitis are allergic, parasitic, and endocrine diseases. In this patient the result of the skin scraping was negative and the pruritus was resolved by treating the overgrowth of bacteria and *Malassezia.* However, the oily seborrhoea and poor haircoat persisted. The owners were advised that a blood test should be performed, as well as an abdominal ultrasound and analyses to measure T_4 and thyroid stimulating hormone (TSH). Ultimately, it was determined that the seborrhoeic dermatitis in this dog was secondary to hypothyroidism.

Case 3

Case presentation

A 13-year-old, intact Dachshund bitch was brought to the clinic with acute prostration. She was not receiving any medication.

Examination revealed haemorrhage of the conjunctiva and the anterior chamber in both eyes, a subcutaneous mass in the right mammary chain, and skin lesions on the abdomen (Fig. 3.1).

Questions

1. What skin lesions do you see in this patient?
2. What could have caused these lesions?
3. Based on the possible differential diagnoses, what diagnostic tests would you perform?

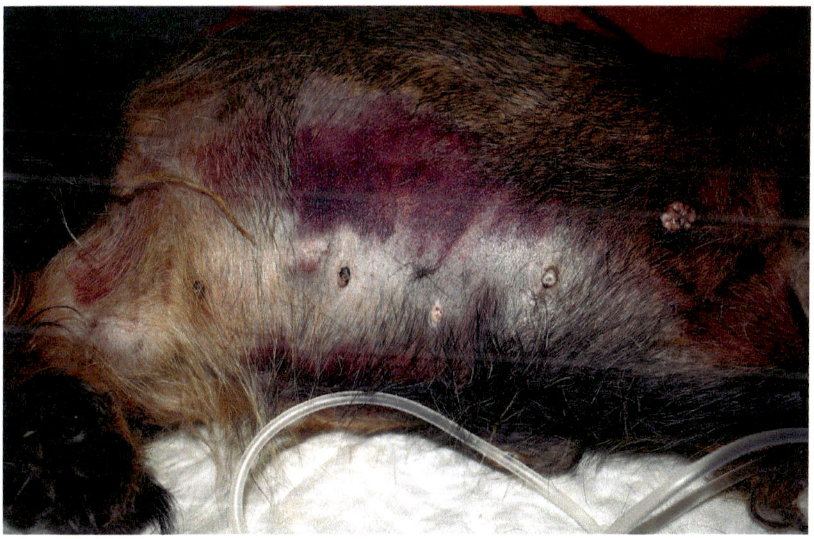

Figure 3.1. Skin lesions on the patient's abdomen.

Answers Case 3

1 What skin lesions do you see in this patient?

The skin lesion is a purpura or a massive haemorrhage in the dermis. While in this case the diagnosis is quite evident given the colour of the skin, in case of doubt a diagnostic technique called diascopy can be used. This involves pressing a glass slide against the skin.

- If the pressure causes the erythematous or purple colour to disappear, the lesion is due to vascular vasodilation.
- If it does not disappear, it is caused by bleeding.

2 What could have caused these lesions?

Haemorrhage in the skin can be caused by trauma, a bleeding disorder, or vasculitis. In this case, the patient showed generalised haemorrhage, suggestive of a coagulation problem.

3 Based on the possible differential diagnoses, what diagnostic tests would you perform?

Because the dog had no clinical history of trauma, blood tests and coagulation tests were performed. The haemogram indicated severe thrombocytopaenia, while secondary coagulation tests were normal. Ultrasonography revealed an ovarian tumour. Some ovarian tumours are oestrogen-producing and can cause spinal aplasia.

Case 4

Case presentation

A 1-year-old guinea pig presented with a pruritic condition that developed after living with a wild rabbit. Scaling was evident, as well as the presence of material adhered to the hair shafts (Fig. 4.1). In the trichogram, the parasite shown in Figure 4.2 was observed.

Questions

1 What parasite is this?
Is its presence related to the wild rabbit?

2 How should it be treated?

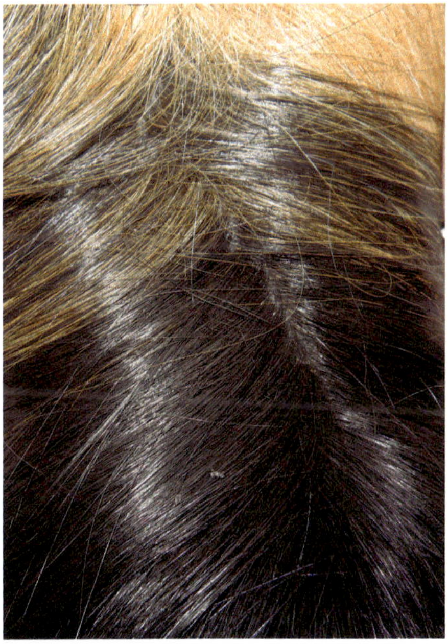

Figure 4.1. Appearance of the hair.

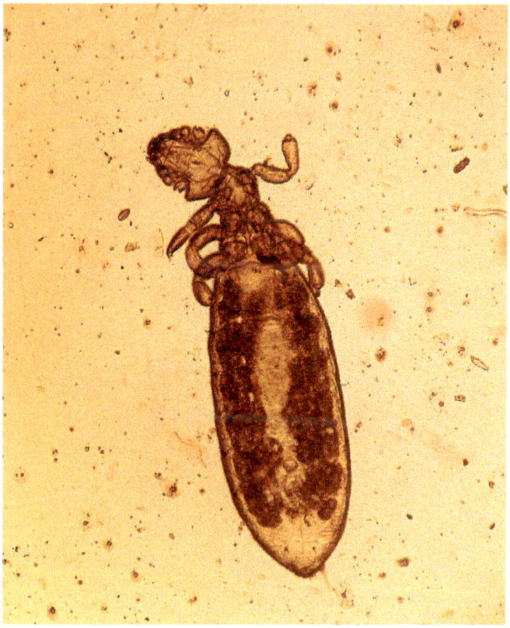

Figure 4.2. Parasite.

Answers to Case 4

1 What parasite is this? Is its presence related to the wild rabbit?

The parasite is *Gliricola porcelli* (the slender guinea pig louse). It is a biting louse that commonly affects guinea pigs. Infestations are usually asymptomatic, but can cause pruritus, alopecia, and a dry, rough haircoat. Diagnosis is established by observing the parasite on the hair shaft under a magnifying glass or microscope.

Contact with the wild rabbit is not likely a relevant factor, since the louse found in wild rabbits is a sucking louse called *Haemodipsus ventricosus.*

2 How should it be treated?

Permethrin or ivermectin can be used for treatment. In this case the patient was treated with topical selamectin (pipette).

Case 5

Case presentation

An intact mongrel dog, aged 6 years and weighing 9 kg, was brought to the clinic for treatment of a nail that had been in poor condition for 3 years. Over this period the problem had improved with antibiotic treatment, but subsequently worsened. The dog previously had leishmaniasis, but the most recent antibody titres were negative. Bacterial culture of the nail was also negative. The patient showed no signs of lameness, and the nail had neither fallen off nor broken, although the animal continually licked the affected digit. Lesions had also recently developed on the face, and improved and worsened in a cyclical manner. The dog was fed with lamb- or salmon-based feed, was in generally good health, and lived with other dogs that had no skin lesions.

The general examination revealed no findings of note. Ulcerative and painful lesions were detected in the lacrimal and labial commissures (Figs. 5.1–5.3), as well as inflammation of the nail bed of the lateral digit of the right forepaw with exudation, pain, and swelling of the adjacent soft tissue (Figs. 5.4 and 5.5).

Cytology of the periungual exudate revealed a purulent pattern. Analysis of a sample taken from the ulcerative lesions revealed the presence of neutrophilic granulocytes with intracellular and extracellular bacteria (cocci).

Questions

1. What problems does this dog have? What are the most likely diagnoses?
2. What diagnostic tests would you perform?

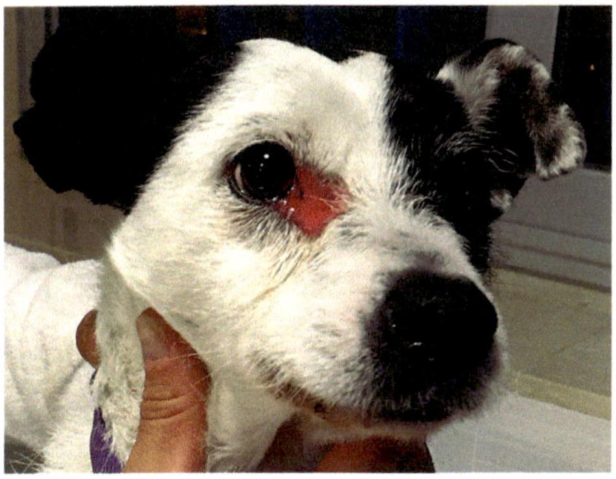

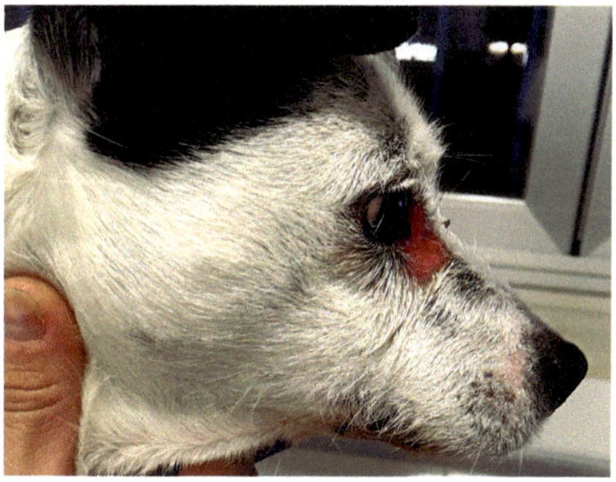

Figures 5.1 and 5.2. Lesions on the patient's face.

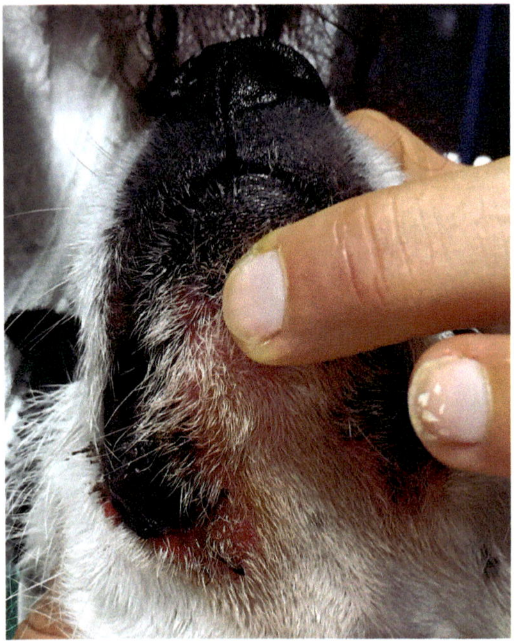

Figure 5.3. Ulceration in the corners of the mouth

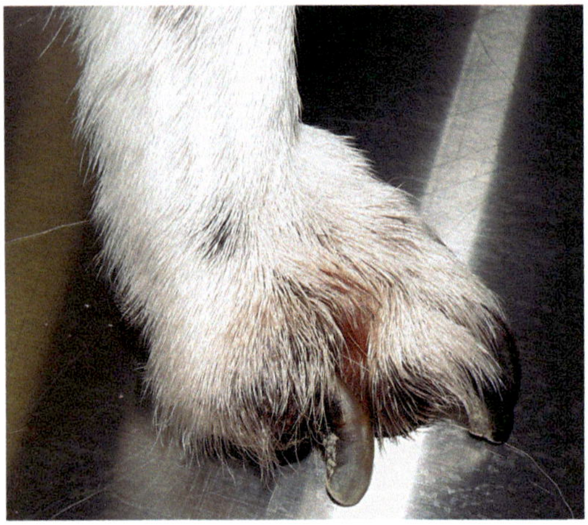

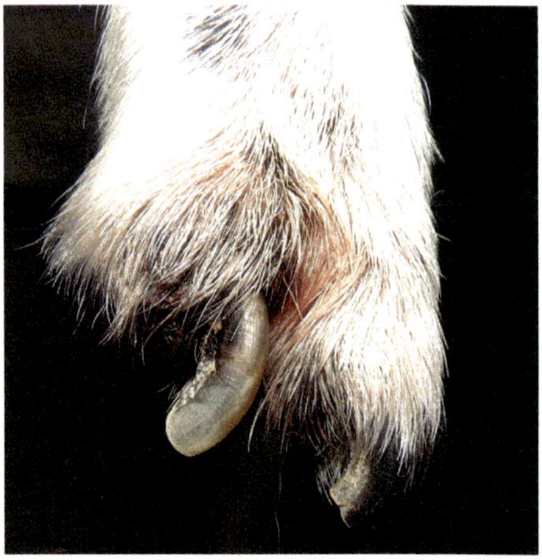

Figures 5.4 and 5.5. Inflammation of the nail bed and adjacent soft tissues.

Answers Case 5

1 What problems does this dog have? What are the most likely diagnoses?

This dog had a paronychia associated with a suppurative process affecting the entire digit, as well as ulcerative lesions at mucocutaneous junctions and chronic leishmaniasis. The inflammation of the digit partially responded to antibiotic treatment.

The following are the most probable differential diagnoses for the process affecting the digit: deep pyoderma with associated paronychia; leishmaniasis; and a neoplasm with secondary infection. In cases of ulcerative lesions in mucocutaneous areas, the differential diagnosis should include mucocutaneous pyoderma, leishmaniasis with an ulcerative pattern, an autoimmune disease (e.g. discoid lupus), and a reaction to a medication.

2 What diagnostic tests would you perform?

Radiography of the affected digit revealed a periosteal reaction in the third phalanx. Culture and antibiogram of the purulent periungual exudate revealed the presence of cephalosporin-sensitive and fluoroquinolone-resistant *Staphylococcus pseudintermedius*. Given the suspicion of osteomyelitis, amputation of the affected digit was recommended. The mucocutaneous lesions were treated with topical fusidic acid. Histopathology of the amputated digit showed subungual inflammation and necrotising suppurative paronychia with periosteal involvement. Immunohistochemical staining for leishmaniasis was negative. Resolution of the mucocutaneous lesions was observed 4 weeks after starting topical antibiotic treatment.

Observations

The most likely cause of a suppurative inflammatory process affecting a single digit is trauma complicated by a secondary bacterial infection. Given that this was a chronic and painful process with bone involvement, and that amputation would not affect locomotion, surgical removal and subsequent analysis of the digit were recommended. Specific stains for leishmaniasis ruled out this disease as the cause of the entire inflammatory process.

Mucocutaneous pyoderma is a syndrome characterised by erythema, inflammation, exudation, erosions, and ulcers of the mucocutaneous junctions, mainly the lips and eyelids. While the pathogenesis of this disease is unknown, bacterial infections are thought to play an important role. However, given the often slow response to antibiotics and frequent recurrences, it has been proposed that mucocutaneous pyoderma may have a more complex immunological basis.

The lesions are usually symmetrical and painful. Depigmentation of the skin can occur in chronic cases. Although the most commonly affected areas are the lips and eyelids, mucocutaneous pyoderma can also affect the nasal plane, prepuce, and perianal region. In this case, the lesions responded well to treatment with topical antibiotics. In case of a poor response, a biopsy should be performed to rule out infectious, immune-mediated, or neoplastic diseases.

Case 6

Case presentation

An intact male Maltese, aged 10 years and weighing 4.25 kg, was brought to the clinic with hair loss on the backs of the thighs and the skin of the abdomen that had begun 1 year earlier. The patient had been receiving 2.5 mg of oral prednisone every 24 hours for several months. Blood tests revealed increased transaminase levels.

Testicular asymmetry was observed in the general examination. Alopecia affected the skin of the abdomen, perineal area, and the base of the tail. Scaling and marked exfoliation of the skin were evident, especially in the perianal area, (Figs. 6.1 and 6.2). Along the prepuce, a linear lesion ran from the tip of the penis to the scrotum (Fig. 6.3).

Questions

1. What type of alopecia does this patient have?
2. What type of lesion is shown in Figure 6.3, and what is it usually caused by?
3. What are the appropriate diagnostic and therapeutic protocols for this patient?

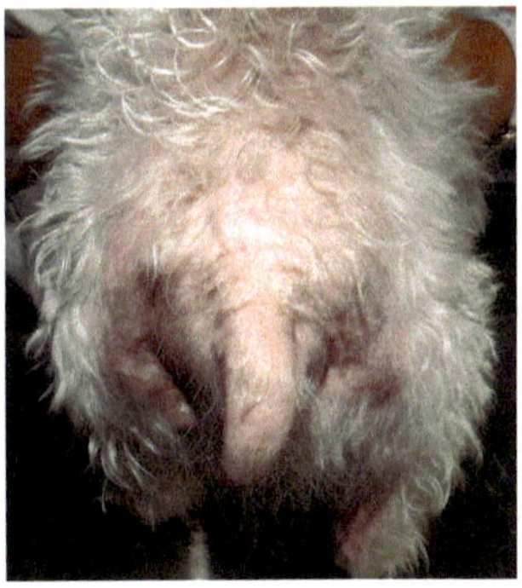

Figure 6.1

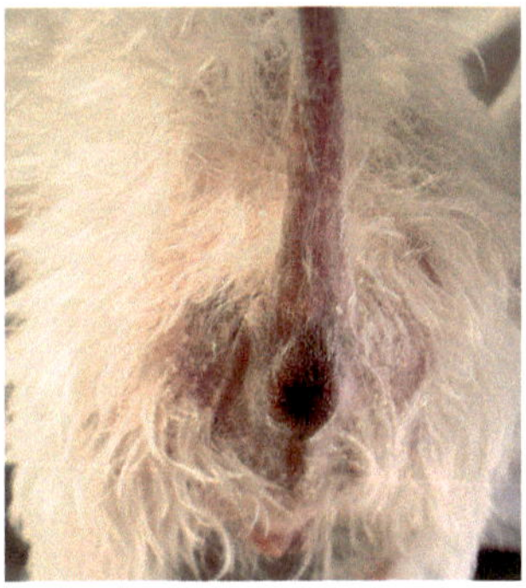

Figure 6.2

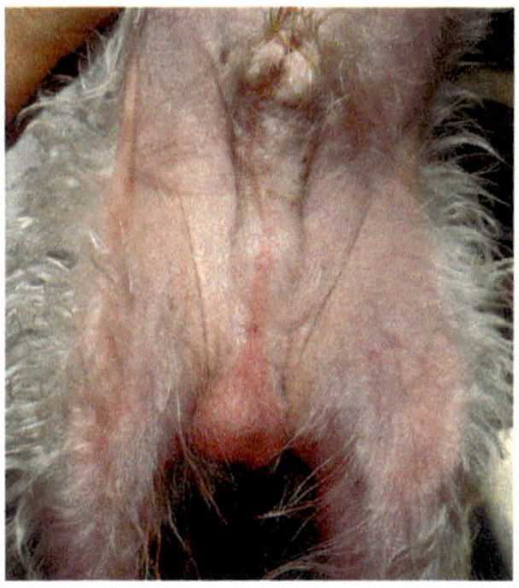

Figure 6.3

Answers Case 6

1 What type of alopecia does this patient have?

The dog has noninflammatory alopecia with severe dehydration of the skin (xerosis).

2 What type of lesion is shown in Figure 6.3, and what is it usually caused by?

The image shows linear preputial dermatosis, which is characterised by a pigmentary alteration that extends linearly from the preputial orifice to the scrotum (Figs. 6.3 and 6.4). While the mechanisms underlying this clinical sign are unknown, it appears to be a specific marker for oestrogen-producing testicular tumours (Sertoli cell tumours of the testicles in males). While interstitial cell tumours can also secrete oestrogen, this is less common. Seminomas rarely secrete hormones. Sertoli cell tumours most commonly occur in the right testicle. This tumour type is usually palpable, and the contralateral testicle is usually atrophied.

Affected dogs may show varying degrees of hyperpigmentation ranging from diffuse hyperpigmentation in alopecic areas to the appearance of macular melanosis (hyperpigmented macules on the perineum and the skin of the abdomen). These hyperpigmented macules are typical of oestrogen-producing tumours (both Sertoli cell and interstitial cell tumours).

3 What are the appropriate diagnostic and therapeutic protocols for this patient?

Chronic administration of prednisone could account for the xerosis and increased transaminase levels. An abdominal ultrasound confirmed the presence of a testicular tumour and liver disease, possibly secondary to glucocorticoid treatment. A gradual decrease in the oral prednisone dose until discontinuation was prescribed, and castration and treatment with emollients and topical moisturisers was recommended.

In the absence of tumour metastasis or oestrogen-induced myelotoxicity, the prognosis for these patients is excellent. The hair grows back around 3 months after castration.

Figure 6.1. Noninflammatory alopecia on the rump and perianal area.

Figure 6.2. Scaling and xerosis at the base of the tail and around the anus.

Figure 6.3. Linear preputial erythema.

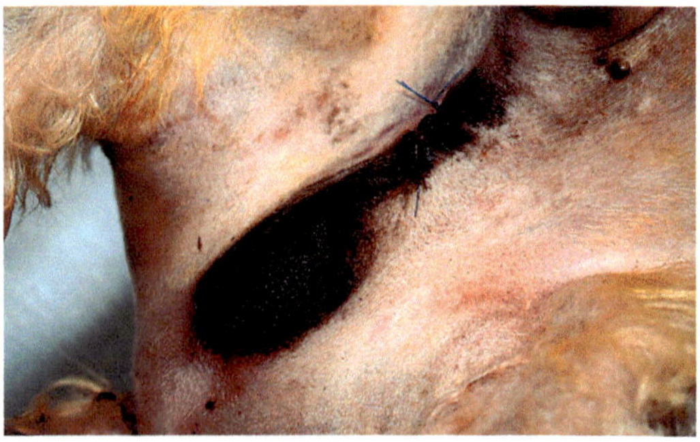

Figure 6.4. Linear preputial erythema in another patient. ▶

Case 7

Case presentation

A 7-year-old Golden Retriever bitch was brought to the clinic with a "blister" on the right hindlimb that had appeared a few months earlier. While the blister appeared not to bother the dog, the owners noticed that it changed size and sometimes colour (turning blue).

A skin nodule with slight erythema was observed in the examination. Fine-needle aspiration of the nodule was performed (Figs. 7.1 and 7.2).

Questions

1 What does the clinical history of this patient suggest?

2 What is the most likely diagnosis of the cytological sample?

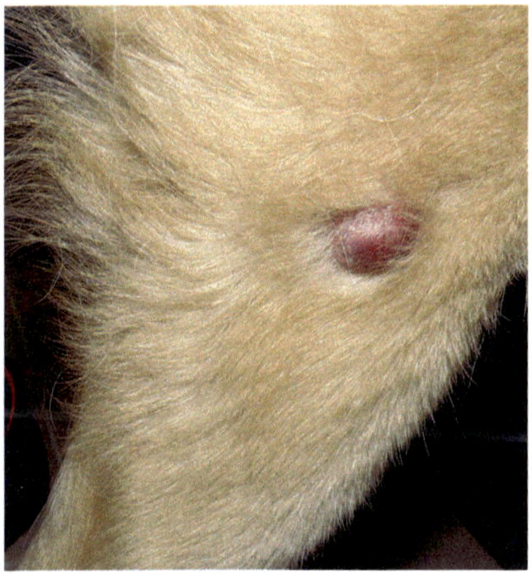

Figure 7.1. Cutaneous nodule on the external aspect of the patient's thigh.

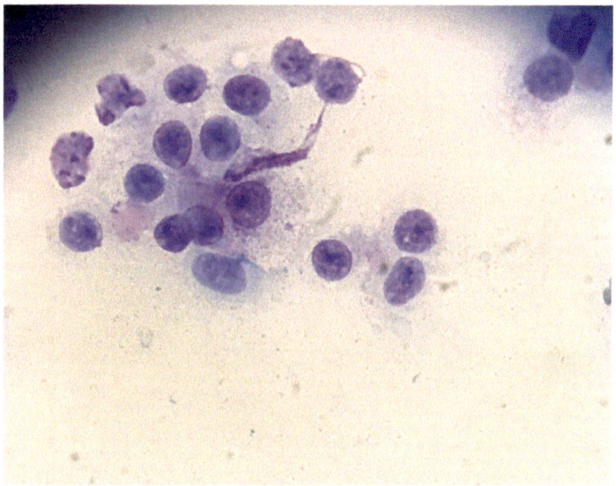

Figure 7.2. Cytological image showing the aspirate extracted from the nodule.

Answers Case 7

1 What does the clinical history of this patient suggest?

In cases involving cutaneous nodules it is important to determine whether the underlying process is inflammatory or neoplastic. The clinical appearance of the lesion can aid diagnosis; heat, redness, and pain are more indicative of an inflammatory process. In this case, we know that this nodule has grown and has undergone changes in colouration, but is not painful. Mast cell tumours are tumours that can change size and colouration and have an inflammatory component, due to the release by tumour cells of vasoactive substances such as histamine and heparin.

2 What is the most likely diagnosis of the cytological sample?

Analysis of the sample reveals a population of round cells with small numbers of eosinophilic granulocytes. The round cells exhibit mild basophilic granulation in the cytoplasm and moderate anisocytosis. This profile is suggestive of a cutaneous round cell neoplasm. Based on the clinical appearance of the tumour and the presence of eosinophils, it is likely a mast cell tumour, but in this case cytology alone is insufficient to establish diagnosis. In some mast cell tumours, rapid staining may not adequately stain the characteristic cytoplasmic granules (Fig. 7.3). Alternatively, the tumour could be a poorly differentiated mast cell tumour or another type of round cell tumour. The following procedures were recommended to the owners of this dog: sentinel lymph node cytology, an abdominal ultrasound to rule out metastasis in the spleen and liver, and aggressive surgery with biopsy to confirm the diagnosis and the complete removal of the tumour.

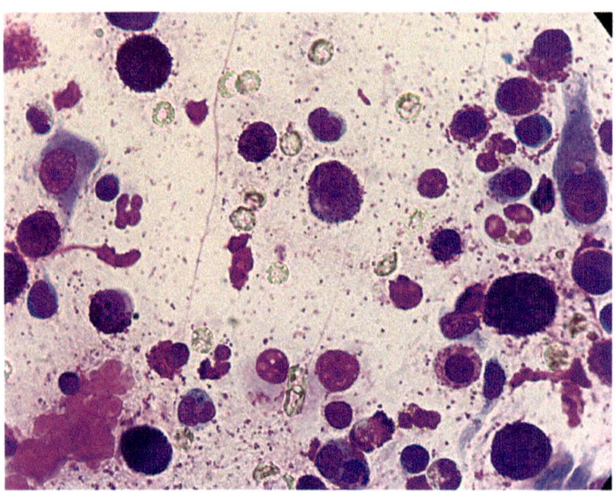

Figure 7.3. Cytological image of a well-differentiated or low-grade cutaneous mastocytoma in which the cytoplasmic granules characteristic of this type of tumour are evident.

Case 8

Case presentation

The patient was a male German Shepherd who had been found and adopted by his owner, and had developed a pyoderma that was complicated with folliculitis and furunculosis. He had been treated with multiple antibiotics as well as oral and topical glucocorticoids. Both the pyoderma and the pruritus had improved significantly, but the owner was worried about skin lesions in the groin area that had not healed, despite treatment with topical creams. The appearance of the lesions and the skin is shown in Figure 8.1.

Questions

1. What lesions can be seen in this dog?
2. What may have caused them?

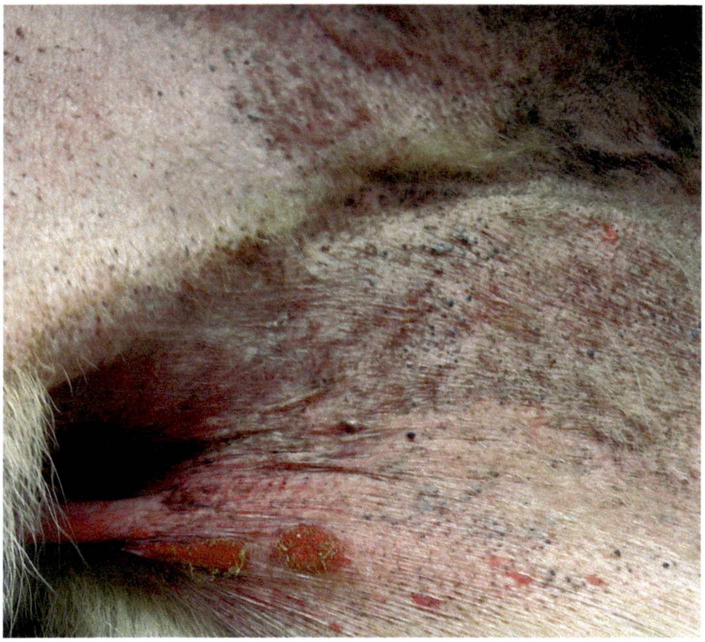

Figure 8.1. Skin lesions on the groin of the patient.

Answers Case 8

1 What lesions can be seen in this dog?

Erosions with scaling, comedones, and milia (Fig. 8.2, arrow).

2 What may have caused them?

These lesions may be due to continued treatment with topical corticosteroids. Topical glucocorticoids cause skin atrophy (thin skin that tends to wrinkle, as if dehydrated), susceptibility to bruising and ecchymosis, seborrhoea, comedones, milia, delayed wound healing, and the appearance of estriae, eschar, and cutaneous calcinosis. Estriae consist of scar tissue, while the term milia describes accumulations of white keratin that resemble comedones but are sealed rather than open, and therefore lack the typical dark colour of comedones (Figs. 8.3 and 8.4).

Topical glucocorticoid treatment was withdrawn and the patient was prescribed washes with chlorhexidine solution to prevent secondary infections. It was advised to allow the skin to recover over 3 to 4 months.

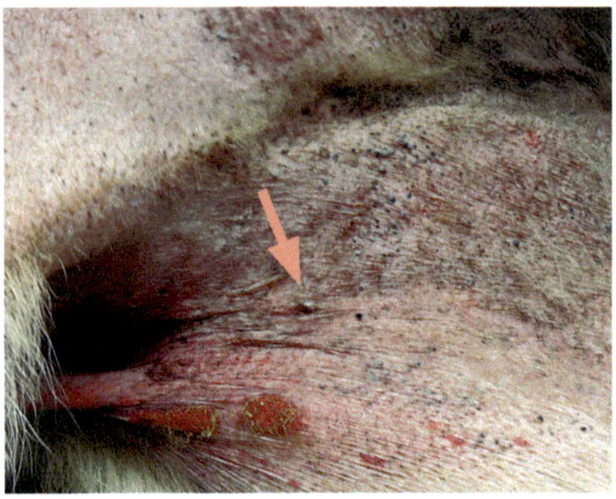

Figure 8.2. Erosions with scaling, comedones, and milia (arrow).

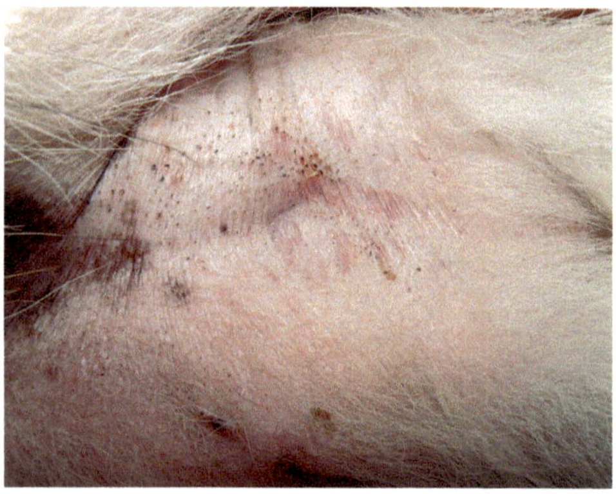

Figure 8.3. Cutaneous estriae.

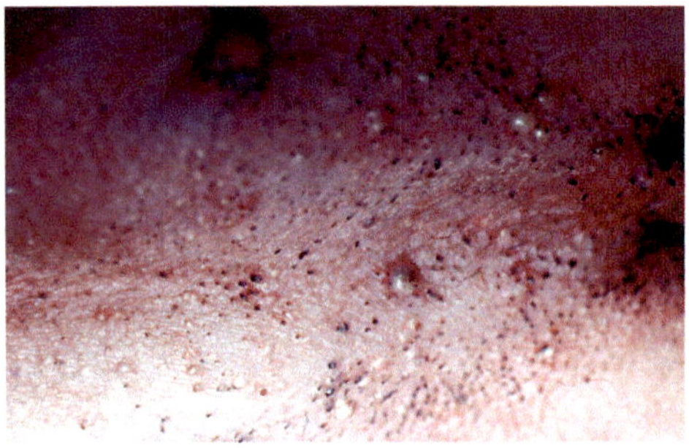

Figure 8.4. Presence of comedones and milia in a dog with iatrogenic hyperadrenocorticism.

Case 9

Case presentation

The patient was an 8-year-old male Golden Retriever, who more than 6 months earlier had developed a fistula between the second and third digits of the left hindlimb. The fistula had not resolved, but had improved following treatment with antibiotics and oral glucocorticoids. The general examination revealed no findings of note. However, in addition to the interdigital fistula, the affected digit was inflamed and swollen (Fig. 9.1).

Exudate cytology (Figs. 9.2–9.4), bacterial culture, and radiography of the digits were performed. Radiography showed an increase in soft tissue density, without bone lesions. *Staphylococcus pseudintermedius* sensitive to cephalosporin and enhanced penicillin was detected in the culture.

Questions

1. What do the cytological images show?
2. What pathology is suggested?

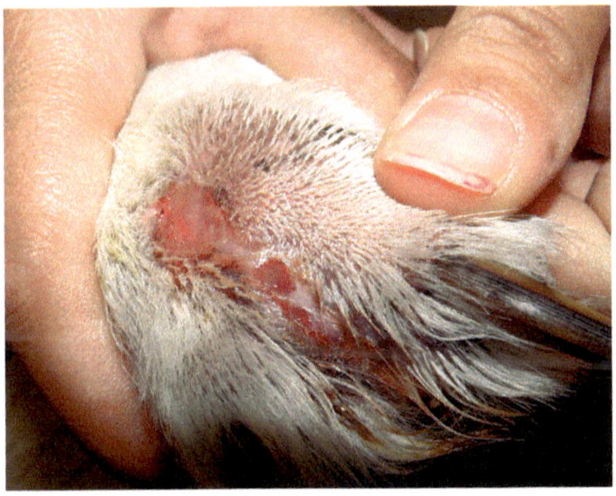

◄ Figure 9.1. Interdigital fistula with inflammation and swelling of the digit.

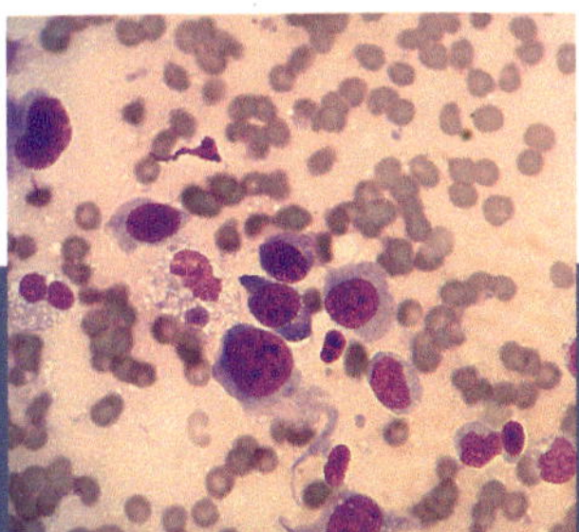

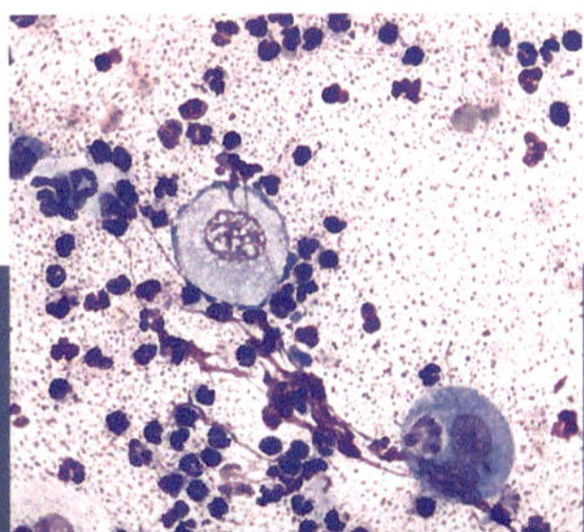

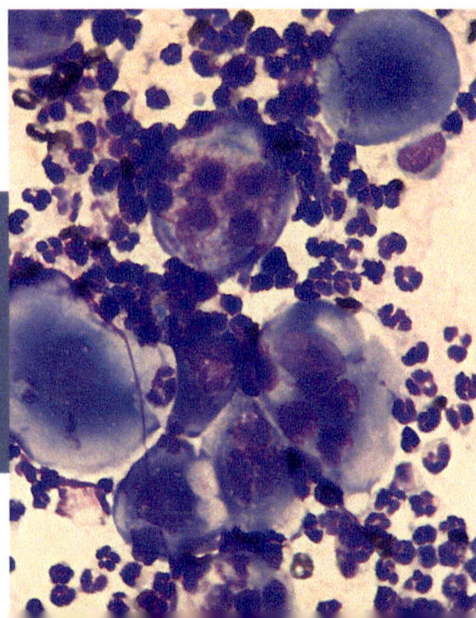

Figures 9.2–9.4. Images of the exudate.

Answers Case 9

1 What do the cytological images show?

The cytology shows squamous epithelial cells with a clear perinuclear halo and a binucleated cell with a prominent nucleolus, as well as a neutrophilic inflammatory infiltrate (Fig. 9.2). Several epithelial cells that have phagocytosed neutrophils can also be seen (Fig. 9.3). Some epithelial cells have an elongated cytoplasm and a fusiform shape ("comet" cells) (Fig. 9.4).

2 What pathology is suggested?

The image is compatible with a well-differentiated squamous cell carcinoma. The main characteristic of squamous cell tumours, from the cytological point of view, is the asynchrony of maturation between cells and between the nucleus and the cytoplasm. Consequently, increases in the cytoplasmic volume are not accompanied by a corresponding reduction in nuclear volume, as occurs during the normal maturation process. Squamous differentiation is characterised by a rounded nucleus and a large, round to polyhedral cytoplasm with angulated borders and variable chromatism, depending on the degree of keratinisation. Colour ranges from blue to pink, and decreases in intensity towards the periphery of the cell.

Atypia is also observed, as evidenced by the presence of nuclei of varying sizes (anisokaryosis), ranging from small to very large, with thick chromatin and multiple nucleoli. Perinuclear vacuolations (halos) and cell cannibalism are also observed.

In some squamous cell carcinomas, cells with tail-like cytoplasmic prolongations ("tadpole" or "comet" cells) can be observed.

Observations

Squamous cell carcinomas are neoplasms of keratinocytes and contain keratin, which can cause an intense secondary pyogranulomatous inflammatory process. This appearance should be taken into account when examining samples of chronic inflammatory processes, in which keratinocytes may exhibit cellular dysplasia induced by inflammation (Fig. 9.5).

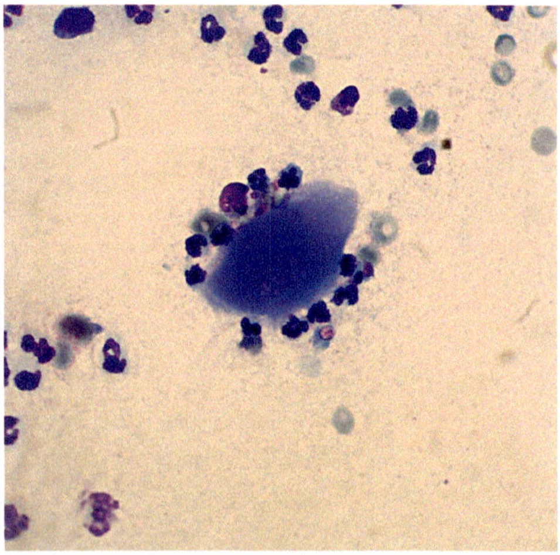

Figure 9.5. Well-differentiated epithelium surrounded by neutrophilic inflammation.

Case 10

Case presentation

A dog was brought for to the veterinary clinic by his owner, who complained that the animal continuously shed large amounts of hair, requiring her to constantly sweep and vacuum the house. The patient, a 5-year-old male mongrel, was healthy and happy, but had persistently shed large tufts of hair over the preceding few months.

The general examination revealed no findings of note, other than massive loss of hair, with no alopecia or other skin lesions (Fig. 10.1).

Questions

1. What can we explain to the owner of this dog?
2. Should the owner be worried?

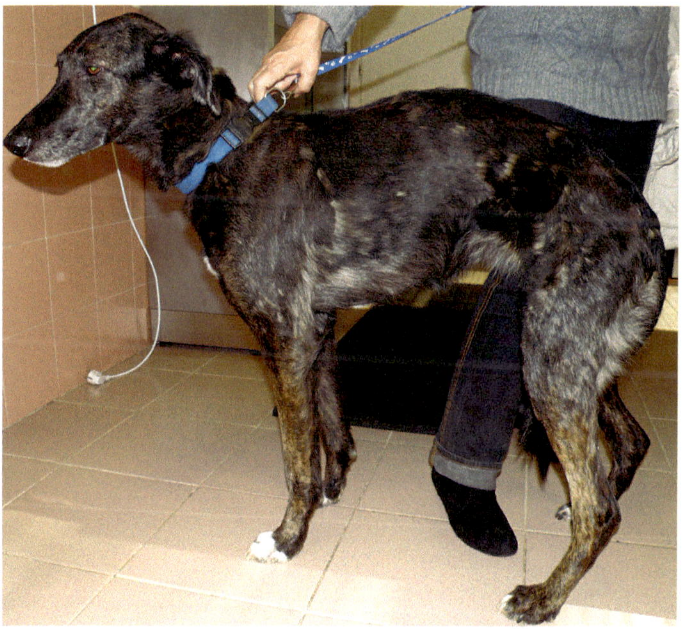

Figure 10.1. Haircoat of the patient, from which tufts of hair are about to fall.

Answers Case 10

1 What can we explain to the owner of this dog?

Excessive physiological moulting is a process that can be worrying to pet owners. Moulting is a genetically programmed cyclical process, whereby hair in telogen phase is shed. Hair loss in dogs and cats is continuous and mosaic in pattern, although in the northern hemisphere, where climatic seasons are well defined, it is more pronounced in spring and autumn. Artificial light and heat in the pet's living environment make these climatic changes less pronounced and favour continuous moulting throughout the year.

2 Should the owner be worried?

Excessive physiological moulting is a normal process. While telogen hairs can be easily manually removed, this does not cause alopecia, and many hairs remain firmly rooted in the skin. The causes of excessive moulting can include changes in photoperiod and ambient temperature, nutritional deficiencies, and states of anxiety or stress (Fig. 10.2). Nordic breeds, the Chow Chow, the Golden Retriever, and the Labrador appear to be predisposed to excessive physiological moulting.

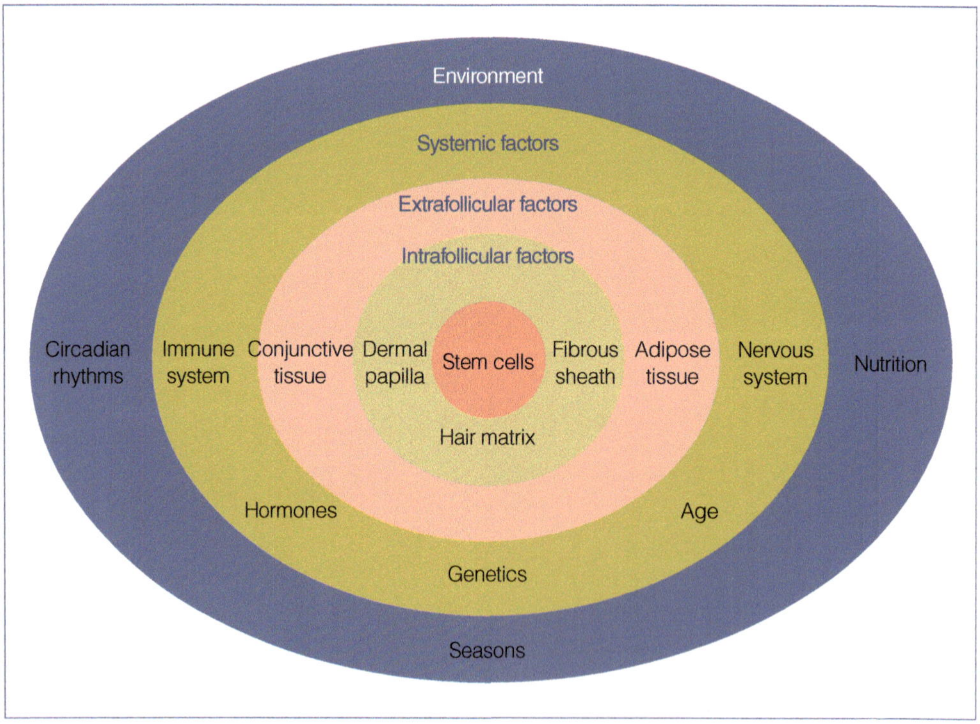

Figure 10.2. Diagram showing the extrinsic and intrinsic factors that can affect the follicular cycle.

Case 11

Case presentation

A 6-year-old Poodle bitch was brought to the clinic for assessment of hair loss from the lateral aspect of the trunk and the rump. She was intact and had been in heat 2 months earlier. According to the owner the dog was healthy, but showed progressive hair loss, which had begun about 1 year earlier. The results of thyroid tests had been normal.

In the general examination, a systolic murmur in the mitral area was detected, as well as noninflammatory symmetrical alopecia of the trunk, tail, and perianal area (Figs. 11.1 and 11.2). Vaginal cytology and a trichogram were performed (Figs. 11.3 and 11.4).

Questions

1. What can be seen in the trichogram and vaginal cytology?
2. What are the main differential diagnoses in this case?

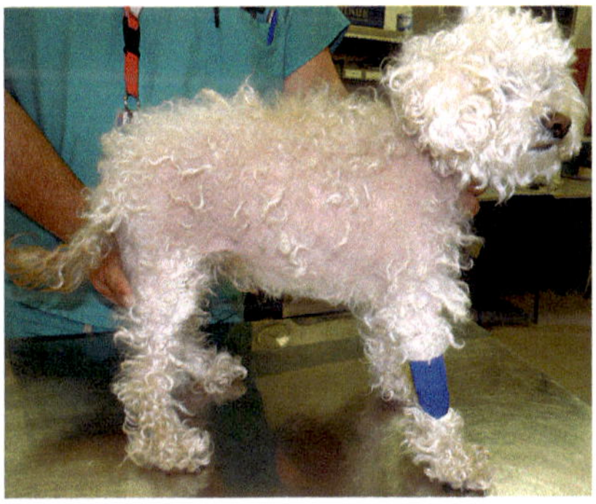

Figure 11.1. Alopecia on the trunk with persistence of secondary hair.

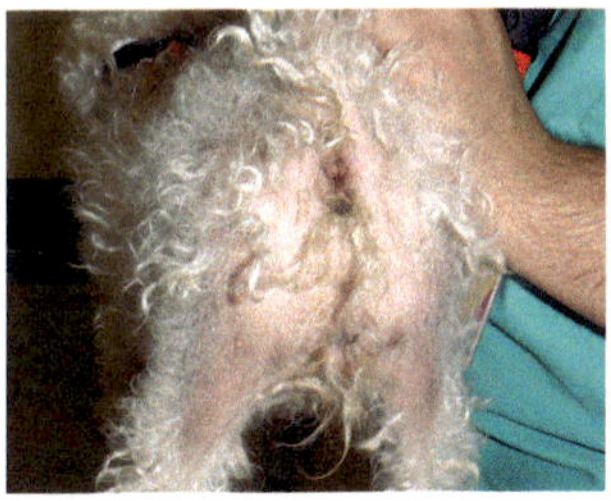

Figure 11.2. Pattern alopecia on the back of the thighs.

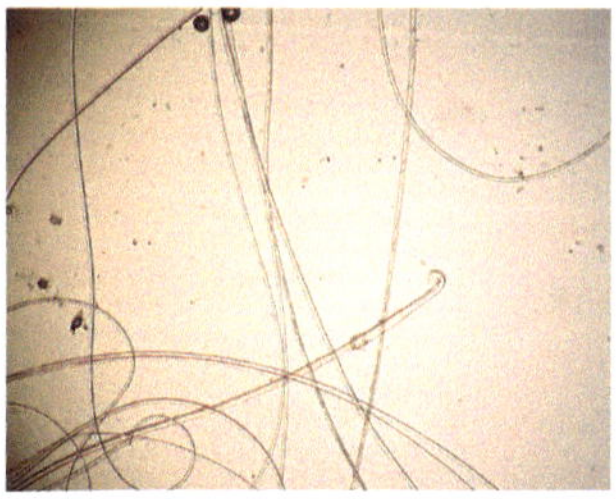

Figure 11.3. Trichogram.

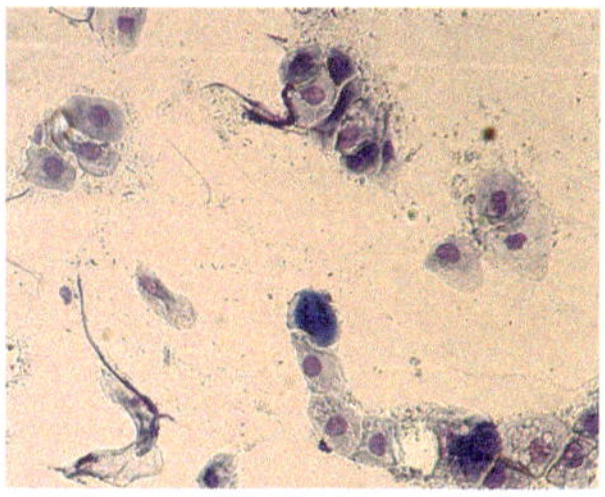

Figure 11.4. Vaginal cytology.

Answers Case 11

1 What can be seen in the trichogram and vaginal cytology?

No parasites are evident in the trichogram, and the appearance of the hair is that of a secondary hair (thin with almost no medullary pigmentation) in telogen phase. The vaginal cytology corresponds to dioestrus.

2 What are the main differential diagnoses in this case?

The differential diagnosis of a middle-aged bitch with generalised noninflammatory alopecia should include the most common endocrinopathies (hypothyroidism, hyperadrenocorticism, and sex hormone imbalance), as well as alopecia X and alopecia due to follicular cycle arrest. In this case, although systemic clinical signs were absent and the oestrous cycle was normal, the patient underwent blood and urine analyses, dynamic tests to rule out hyperadrenocorticism, and an abdominal ultrasound. The results of all these tests were normal, and the owners were informed that the patient may have alopecia X.

Observations

Alopecia X is an acquired, progressive, noninflammatory alopecia that mainly affects thick-haired dog breeds and the miniature Poodle. Its aetiology is unknown, although a hereditary component has been proposed. There is no sexual predisposition and hair loss begins between 1 and 10 years of age. Its clinical appearance is similar to that of endocrine alopecia, with the progressive development of a dry, dull haircoat, and loss of primary hair. The first areas affected by alopecia are areas of friction, the tail, and the caudomedial aspects of the thighs. Primary hair is progressively lost from the trunk, with secondary hair remaining, lending the appearance of a puppy coat. Affected dogs are generally in good condition, and show no signs of systemic disease.

Diagnosis is reached by exclusion, after ruling out other processes such as Cushing's syndrome, hypothyroidism, sexual hormone imbalance, cyclic flank alopecia, and follicular dysplasias. In some breeds such as the Samoyed, sebaceous adenitis should also be considered.

Ovariohysterectomy or castration are the treatments of choice in intact dogs, after which growth of permanent or temporary hair is seen in 50 % to 75 % of cases. If neutering is ineffective, or if alopecia recurs 1 or 2 years after neutering, the treatment of choice is melatonin (3–9 mg orally every 8–12 hours for 3–4 months). Between 30 % and 40 % of dogs respond to melatonin, which has few side effects.

In the present case, a skin biopsy taken during neutering was used to confirm the diagnosis.

Case 12

Case presentation

The patient, a male Greyhound of 10 years of age, was brought for consultation with warts on the skin of the sternum (Fig. 12.1). The owner was very worried.

Questions

1. What does the appearance of the warts suggest?
2. What is the prognosis for this lesion?

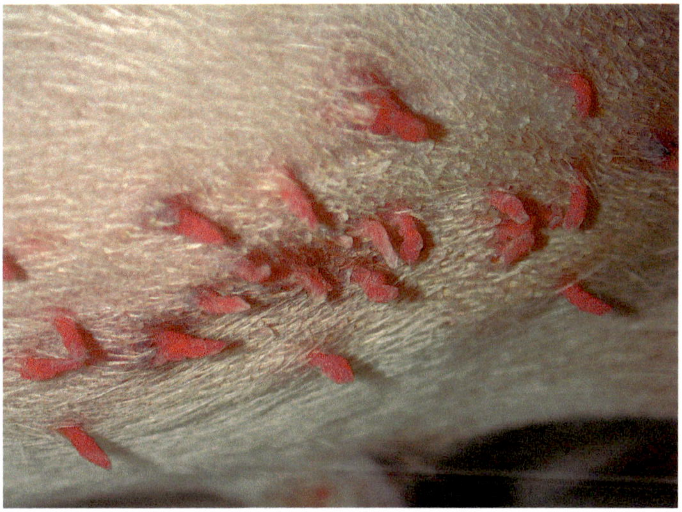

Figure 12.1. Wart-like growths on the skin of the sternum.

Answers Case 12

1 What does the appearance of the warts suggest?

Cutaneous excrescence or fibrovascular papilloma is a benign growth of fibrovascular origin and is usually a response of the skin to repeated trauma. It is rare, and generally affects middle-aged and elderly dogs of large and giant breeds.

The characteristic lesions are firm, pedunculated growths of 1–2 cm in length and a few millimetres in diameter (Fig. 12.2).

Larger lesions may ulcerate. They are most often located on the sternum, bony prominences, and the trunk.

Histopathology reveals a hyperplastic epidermis surrounding a central core of vascularised connective tissue.

2 What is the prognosis for this lesion?

These are benign non-neoplastic lesions, and do not usually require treatment. Lesions that ulcerate can be surgically removed by laser or cryosurgery. The prognosis is good, given the non-neoplastic nature of these lesions.

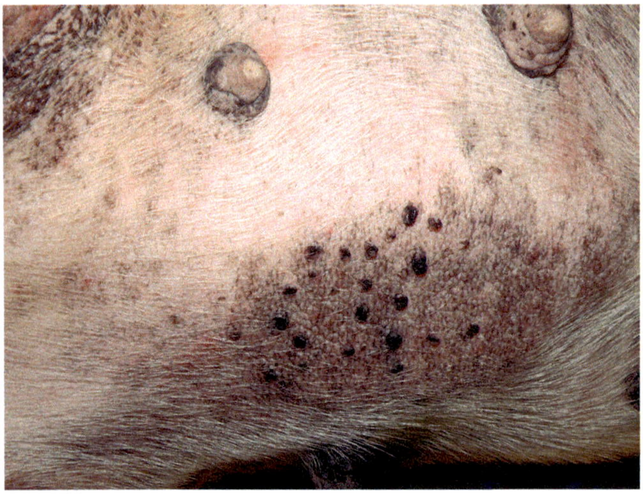

Figure 12.2. Fibrovascular papilloma on the skin of the sternum of a Carlino.

Case 13

Case presentation

An intact male Bull Terrier of 4 years of age was brought to the clinic with a lesion on the nasal bridge (Fig. 13.1). The dog was in good condition and appeared unperturbed by the lesion.

Questions

1. What lesions are observed on the skin?
2. What may have caused them?

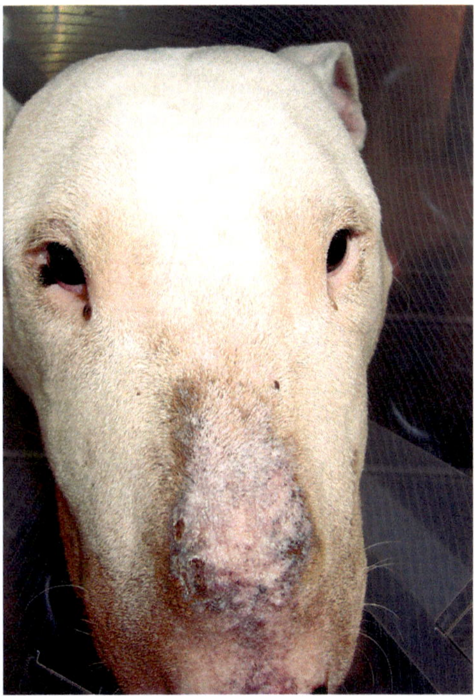

Figure 13.1. Lesion on the nasal bridge.

Answers Case 13

1 What lesions are observed on the skin?

The lesion on the nasal bridge consists of an apparent thickening of the skin, with comedones. No inflammatory lesions (erythema, exudation, etc.) are evident, except for a small crust. The appearance of the lesion is that of a cutaneous callus.

2 What may have caused them?

A callus is a round or oval hyperkeratotic plaque (an increase in the thickness of the corneal layer of the epidermis) that develops on bony prominences or dependent areas. Classic locations include the elbows, tarsals, and sternum. Calluses are a normal response to trauma, ischaemia, or chronic inflammation of the skin. In many cases, repeated trauma gives rise to a very painful secondary pyoderma (Figs. 13.2–13.4).

The presence of calluses on the nasal bridge of this patient is typical of the breed in question. These dogs usually sleep with the bridge of the nose resting on a surface, and exert pressure on this area when playing. This chronic trauma causes calluses to form on the skin.

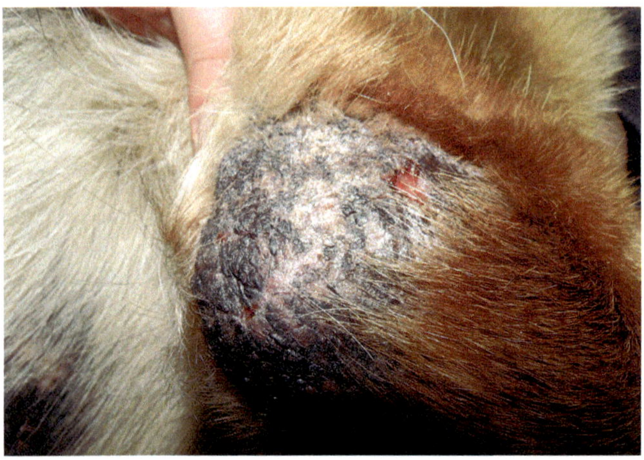

Figure 13.2. Skin callus on the elbow, with superficial pyoderma.

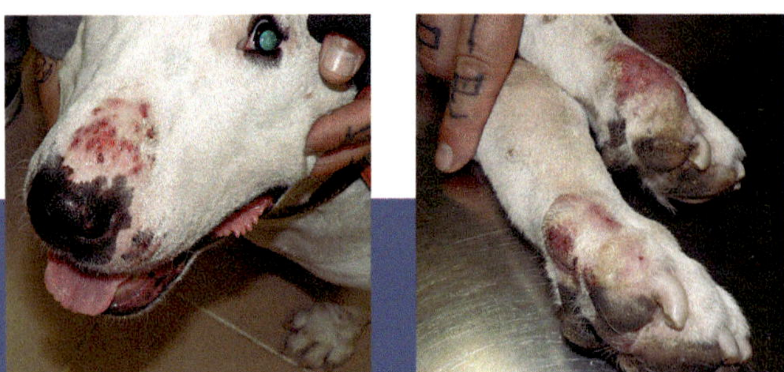

Figures 13.3 and 13.4. Nodular lesions with haemorrhagic and purulent exudate on the nasal bridge and bony prominences of the digits of a Bull Terrier.

Case 14

Case presentation

A 2-month-old male kitten that had been found in the street was brought to the clinic with a hairless spot on the face that appeared not to bother him (Fig. 14.1). The appearance of the lesion, as viewed under a Wood's lamp, is shown in Figure14.2.

Questions

1 What type of lesion is this?

2 What other diagnostic tests can be performed?

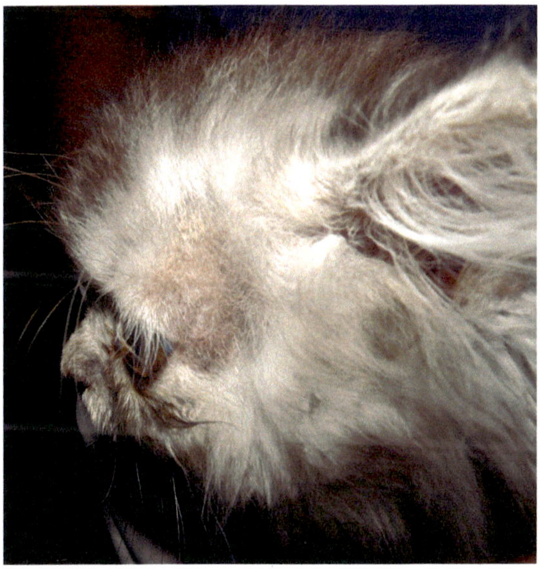

Figure 14.1. Alopecia in the preauricular area of the patient.

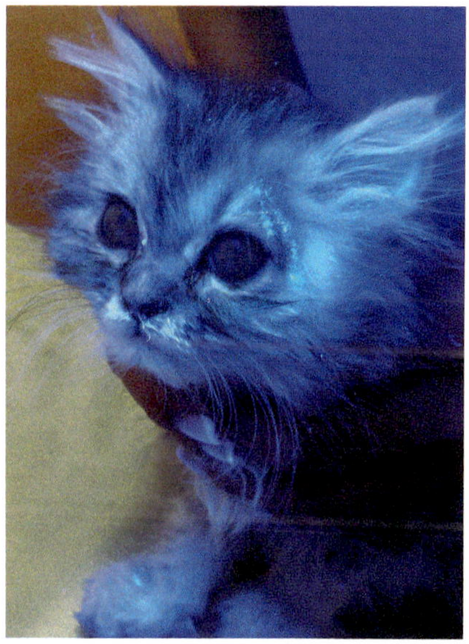

Figure 14.2. Examination of the patient using a Wood's lamp.

Answers Case 14

1 What type of lesion is this?

Everything indicates that the patient has a dermatophytosis. Although the exact prevalence of fluorescence under a Wood's lamp in cats with dermatophytosis is unknown, it is over 50 %. As such, a Wood's lamp is a useful screening tool in cats with alopecia.

The Wood's lamp emits ultraviolet radiation at a wavelength of 320–400 nm that penetrates to the dermis. Certain substances react by absorbing this energy in the form of electromagnetic radiation and emitting it almost instantaneously (within nanoseconds) at a different wavelength, which is visible to the human eye. This phenomenon is known as fluorescence.

In human medicine, the Wood's lamp is used in the diagnosis of many dermatological pathologies (vitiligo, pityriasis versicolor, pityriasis alba, erythrasma, pseudomonas infections, melanoma) and even as a diagnostic tool in internal medicine (porphyria).

The positive fluorescence is apple-green or bluish-green in colour (Fig. 14.2). Only the diaphysis of the hair emits fluorescence. The lamp should be used with magnification in a dark place, and should be held close to the skin (4–10 cm) (Fig. 14.3).

2 What other diagnostic tests can be performed?

The most commonly used tests in the diagnosis of dermatophytosis in cats are physical examination, examination with a Wood's lamp, direct examination of fluorescent hairs, and fungal culture.

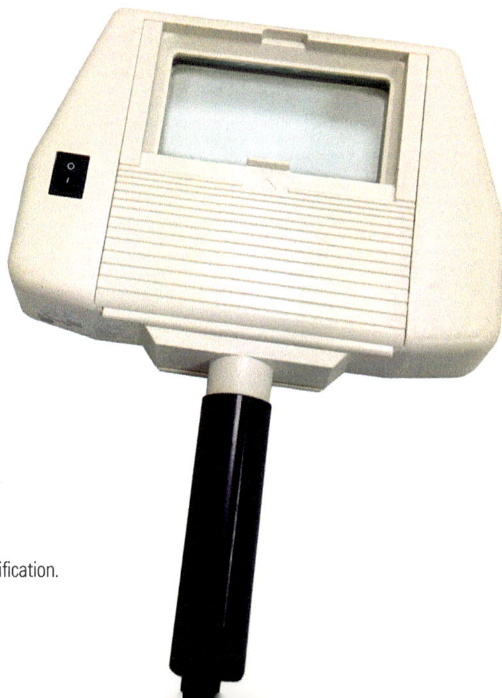

Figure 14.3. Wood's lamp with magnification.

Case 15

Case presentation

A 7-month-old male Pinscher was brought to the veterinary clinic for assessment of "lumps" on the ears that had appeared 2 weeks earlier. Several days later they also appeared on the eyelid (Figs. 15.1 and 15.2). The general condition of the animal was excellent, and he appeared unperturbed by the lesions.

Questions

1 What does this type of lesion suggest?

2 What pathologies should be included in the differential diagnosis?

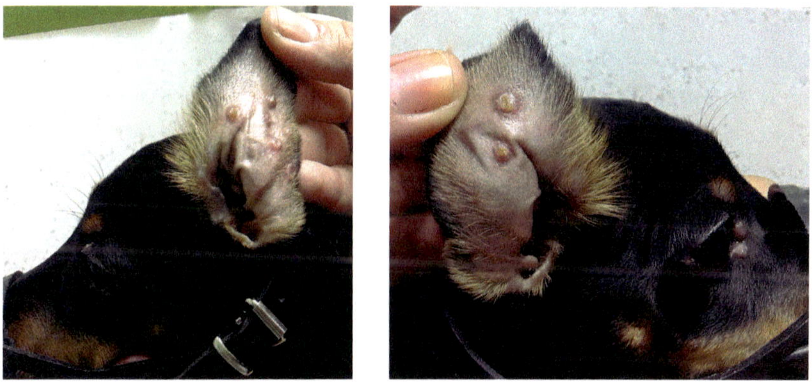

Figures 15.1 and 15.2. Papulonodular lesions on the pinnae and the right eyelid.

Answers Case 15

1 What does this type of lesion suggest?

The lesions observed on the pinna of this puppy are characteristic of the papular pattern associated with leishmaniasis. This is not an inoculation chancre, since in dogs leishmaniasis is always visceral (i.e. does not have an exclusively cutaneous form).

The papular pattern of leishmaniasis is characterised by the presence of persistent papules located in areas with little hair, such as the inner aspect of the pinna, the nasal bridge, the perianal region, and the ventral abdomen. The papules or nodules are firm and slightly erythematous, with a light brown, scaly surface and a slightly umbilical shape (Figs. 15.1–15.3). These types of lesions are neither painful nor pruritic.

These lesions appear to correspond to multiple inoculations with the parasite, and are associated with a good immune response. Affected patients show a low parasitic load, positive skin test results, low serum titre levels, and a good treatment response.

In this case, lesion cytology revealed the presence of a granulomatous inflammatory infiltrate with *Leishmania infantum* amastigotes within the macrophages (Fig. 15.4).

2 What pathologies should be included in the differential diagnosis?

The differential diagnosis of papulonodular lesions in a puppy should include atypical infections, fungal mycetomas, nodular myiasis, eosinophilic granulomas, histiocytoma, and mastocytoma.

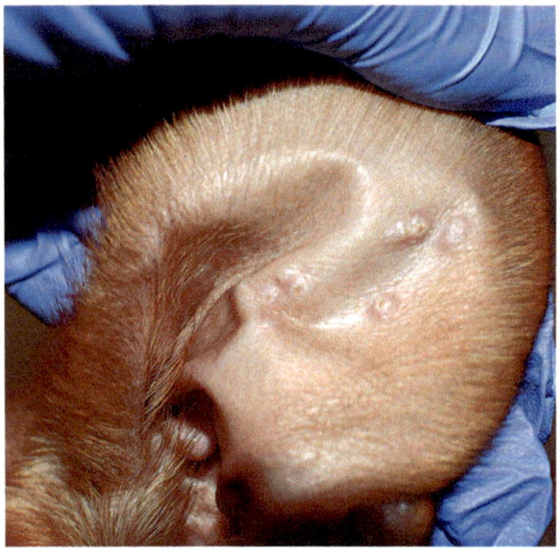

Figure 15.3. Firm papulonodular lesions with a scaly, yellow-brown surface and an umbonate shape typical of the papular presentation of canine leishmaniasis.

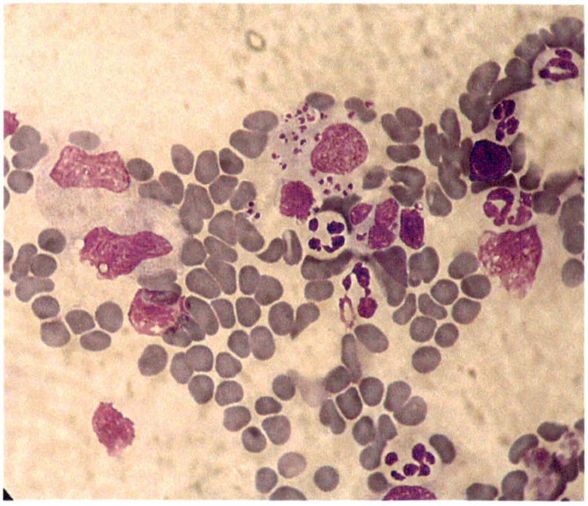

Figure 15.4. Lesion cytology showing amastigotes of *Leishmania infantum* inside a macrophage.

Case 16

Case presentation

The owners of a 4-year-old, intact Yorkshire Terrier bitch reported discolouration of the lower lip that had appeared a few months earlier. The owners had not attributed much significance to the lesion, but then noticed a few weeks prior to the consultation that the discolouration had begun to affect the muzzle. An antibiotic cream had had no effect. While the dog appeared unperturbed by the lesion, the owners were very worried.

The general examination of the bitch revealed no findings of significance. Peribucal depigmentation was observed with erythema on the rostral part of the muzzle, but no loss of anatomical architecture and no ulcers, fissures, or crusts (Figs. 16.1–16.4). The distribution of the lesions was relatively symmetrical.

Question

1 What is the differential diagnosis of this type of lesion in this location?

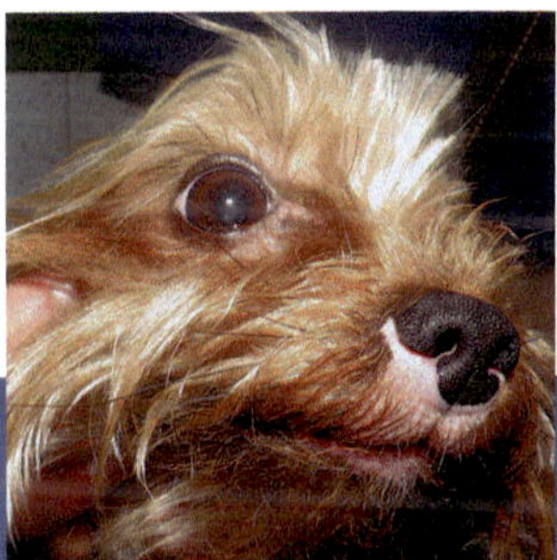

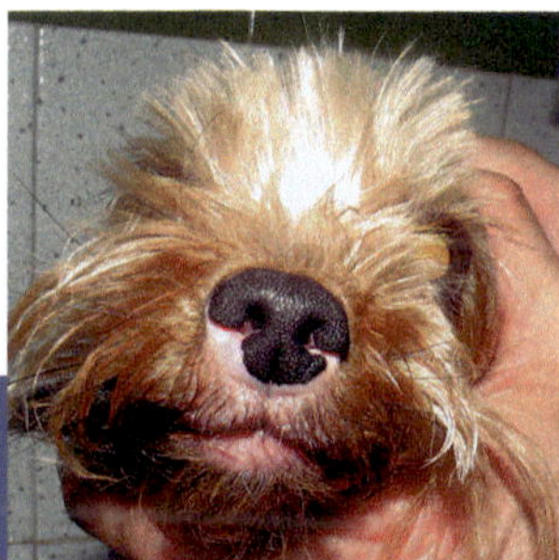

Figures 16.1 and 16.2. Depigmentation and erythema around the mouth and on the rostral aspect of the muzzle.

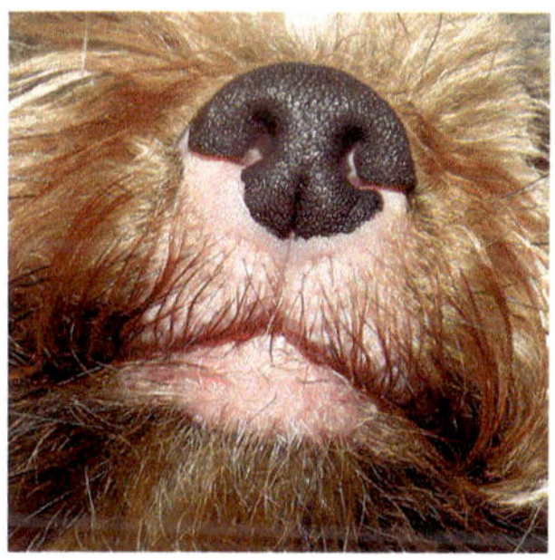

Figure 16.3. Detail of muzzle depigmentation; the normal architecture of the muzzle is maintained.

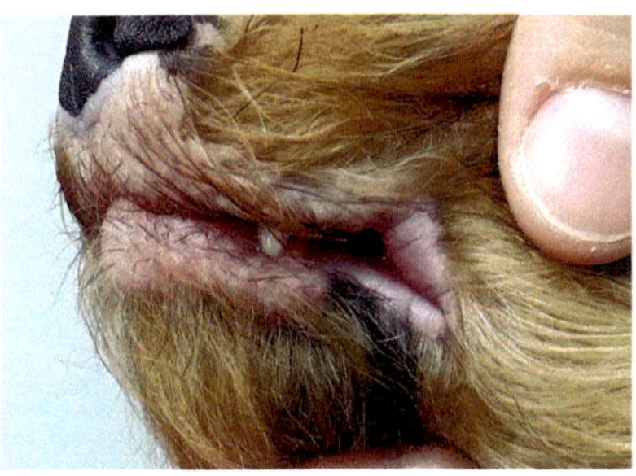

◀ Figure 16.4. Peribucal depigmentation.

Answer Case 16

1 What is the differential diagnosis of this type of lesion in this location?

Like hyperpigmentation, depigmentation of the skin is usually an indicator of inflammation. In addition to depigmentation, inflammatory processes that affect the muzzle can involve ulcers, crusts, and loss of the normal architecture.

The most common causes of inflammation of the muzzle with ulceration are discoid lupus and other autoimmune diseases, mucocutaneous pyoderma, leishmaniasis, uveodermatologic syndrome, and epitheliotropic lymphoma. This patient presented with only depigmentation and erythema.

The most likely differential diagnoses in this case are hereditary nasal depigmentation of Nordic breeds and the Labrador Retriever (snow or winter nose) and vitiligo. The distribution of the lesions in this case is typical of vitiligo.

Observations

Vitiligo is an immune-mediated disease that affects the melanocytes, resulting in depigmentation of the skin and hair. Predisposed breeds include the Rottweiler, Boxer, German Shepherd, and Belgian Shepherd. Histological examination reveals normal skin, except for a lack of melanocytes. The cause of vitiligo is unknown, and there is no effective veterinary treatment, although some cases can resolve spontaneously.

Case 17

Case presentation

The clinical appearance of the patient, a 2-year-old male Persian cat, is shown in Figures 17.1 and 17.2. Prior to the appearance of the lesions, he had received long-term treatment with injectable glucocorticoids for an ophthalmic process. A skin biopsy revealed perivascular hyperplastic dermatitis with follicular keratosis. No parasites, bacterial agents, or fungi were detected, and PAS staining was negative. The cat had not responded to antibiotic treatment and had mild pruritus.

Questions

1 What are the main pathologies that should be included in the differential diagnosis in this case?

2 What diagnostic tests should be performed?

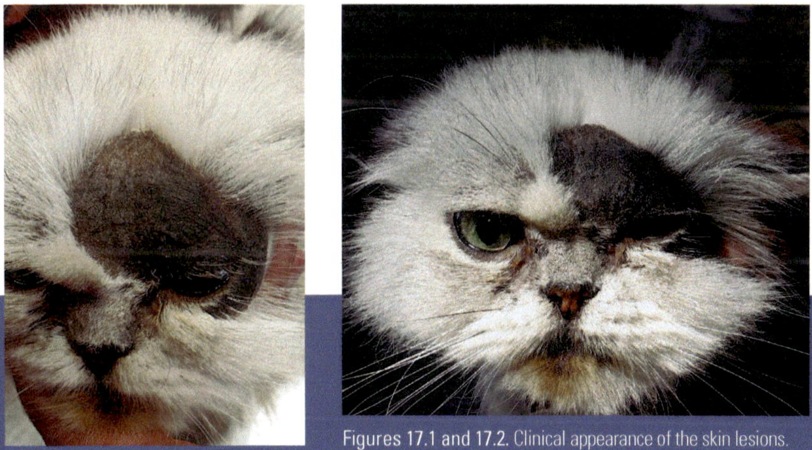

Figures 17.1 and 17.2. Clinical appearance of the skin lesions.

Answers Case 17

1 What are the main pathologies that should be included in the differential diagnosis in this case?

The most salient features in this case are that the patient is a young Persian cat that has undergone prolonged glucocorticoid treatment. The patient's lesions consist of focal nonsymmetrical alopecia with hyperpigmentation and seborrhoea. Inflammatory lesions with follicular keratosis are observed in the biopsy. Based on the patient's clinical history, clinical signs, and biopsy results, the differential diagnosis should include the following:

- Dermatophytosis.
- Demodicosis.
- Superficial pyoderma.
- Viral dermatosis.

2 What diagnostic tests should be performed?

The following diagnostic tests were performed: a bacterial culture, which was negative, and a dermatophyte culture (DTM), which was positive for *Microsporum canis*. The cat showed a good response to oral itraconazole treatment (Fig. 17.3).

Observations

Persian cats can be asymptomatic carriers of dermatophytes. These infections can manifest clinically in immunosuppressed animals. Although the trichogram, biopsy, and PAS staining were negative, a DTM culture was recommended given the strong suspicion of dermatophytosis. It is important to note that skin biopsies should ideally be sent to anatomopathologists familiar with veterinary dermatology.

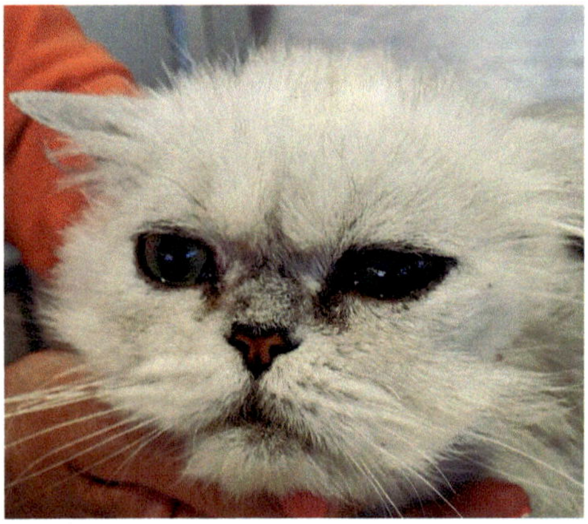

Figure 17.3. Appearance of the cat after 4 weeks of treatment with oral itraconazole.

Case 18

Case presentation

A 2.5-month-old puppy with generalised pruritus was brought for consultation by his owners. Areas of alopecia with some erythema were observed in the thoracolumbar area, as well as small pustules on one of the pinnae (Figs. 18.1–18.3). The animal had been fitted with an insecticidal collar, but the pruritus had persisted.

Questions

1. What could be the cause of this puppy's lesions?
2. What diagnostic tests would be indicated?
3. Could the dog be allergic?

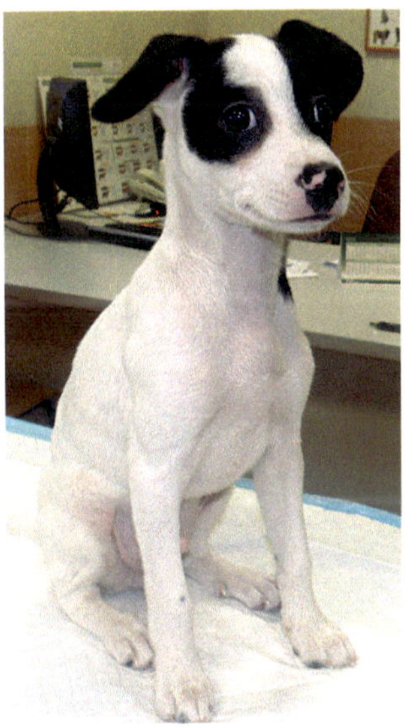

Figure 18.1. Patient with generalised pruritus. Mild erythema is evident on the ventral aspect of the neck and on the skin of the abdomen.

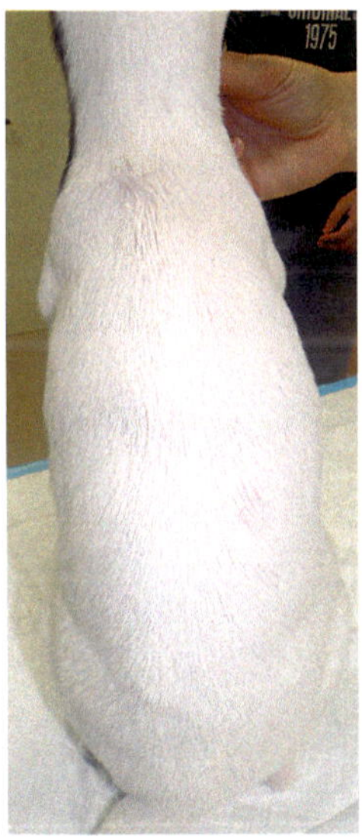

Figure 18.2. Mild hypotrichosis and erythema on the back of the patient.

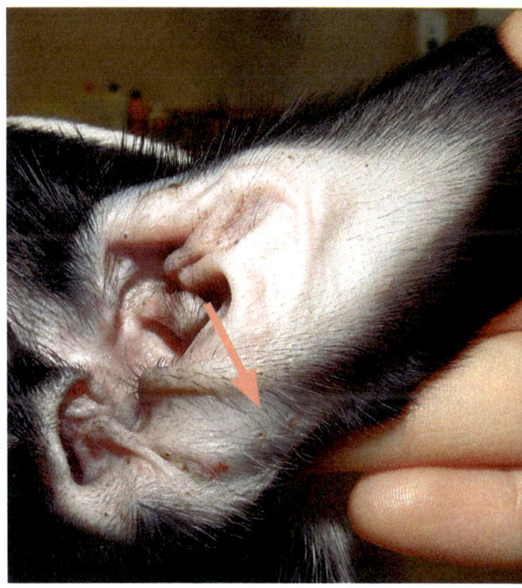

Figure 18.3. Pustular lesions (arrow) on the pinna.

Answers Case 18

1 What could be the cause of this puppy's lesions?

Pruritus in puppies is usually caused by parasites, either external or internal (ascaris). In the case of this puppy, the dorsal distribution suggested parasitisation by *Cheyletiella*, or the presence of fleas.

2 What diagnostic tests would be indicated?

The diagnostic tests indicated for puppies with pruritus are serial coprological analyses and skin brushing and scraping. In this case, while examining and combing the patient to obtain diagnostic material, several fleas jumped onto the examination table.

The pustular lesion on the pinna was a bacterial infection, which did not affect the hair, known as impetigo. Impetigo in puppies can be associated with malnutrition, parasites, or poor sanitary conditions in general (Fig. 18.4).

3 Could the dog be allergic?

It is unlikely that the dog is atopic or has a food intolerance, since these pathologies generally affect dogs from 6 months of age.

The puppy was treated with an antiparasitic pipette and the impetigo resolved once the flea infestation was eliminated.

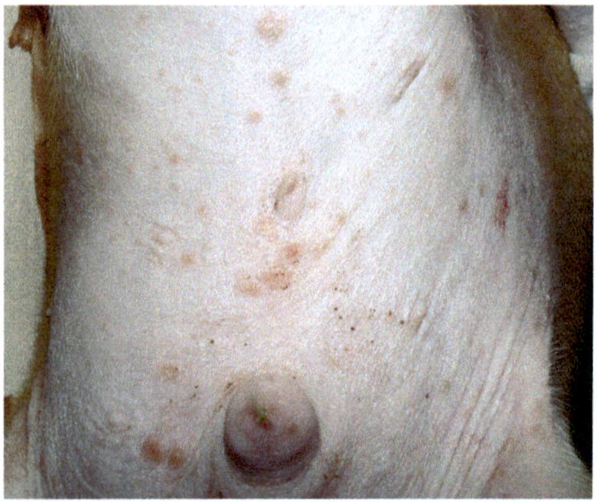

Figure 18.4. Impetigo on the abdominal skin of a puppy.

Case 19

Case presentation

The patient, a 4-year-old Saint Bernard dog, had gone to the beach with his owners several months earlier. From that moment he began to insistently and desperately scratch his right ear. Subsequently, several lesions appeared on the face and elbows. Figures 19.1 and 19.2 show the appearance of the lesions on the pinnae and face of the patient.

Question

1 Can beach sand cause allergic contact dermatitis?

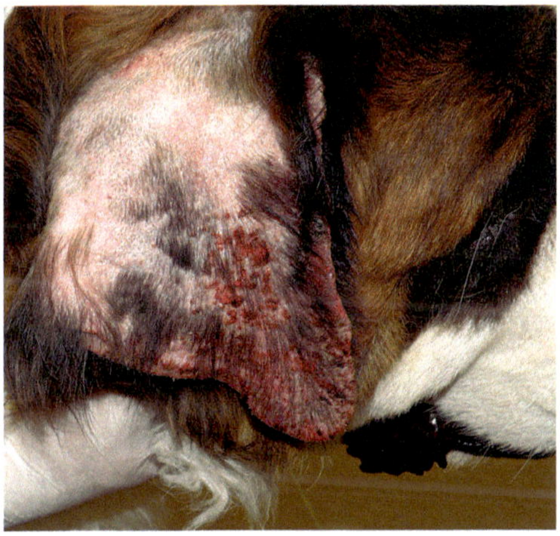

Figure 19.1. Alopecia, erythema, crusted papular lesions, and excoriation on the pinna.

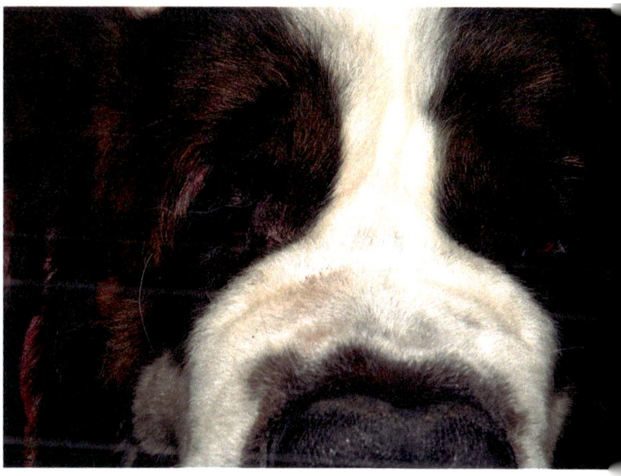

Figure 19.2. Alopecia and erythema on the eyelids on the same side of the face as the lesions of the pinna.

Answer Case 19

1 Can beach sand cause allergic contact dermatitis?

This patient had very intense, subacute pruritus affecting the pinnae and elbows. The following are the most likely differential diagnoses:

- Allergic contact dermatitis.
- Dermatitis due to *Malassezia*.
- Sarcoptic mange.

The distribution of the lesions (pinnal margin, elbows) was highly indicative of sarcoptic mange. Luckily, sarcoptic mites were detected in the skin scraping. Even if the scraping had been negative, treatment for sarcoptic mange would have been indicated (Fig. 19.3). It is possible that the animal had already acquired the parasite before going to the beach and that rolling in the sand was secondary to the intense pruritus caused by the mite.

Scrapings were obtained from the margin of the pinna and the elbow, the sites at which the *Sarcoptes scabiei* mite is most commonly found.

The dog was treated with selamectin (pipette) and glucocorticoids at anti-inflammatory doses for 5 days, with good response (Fig. 19.4).

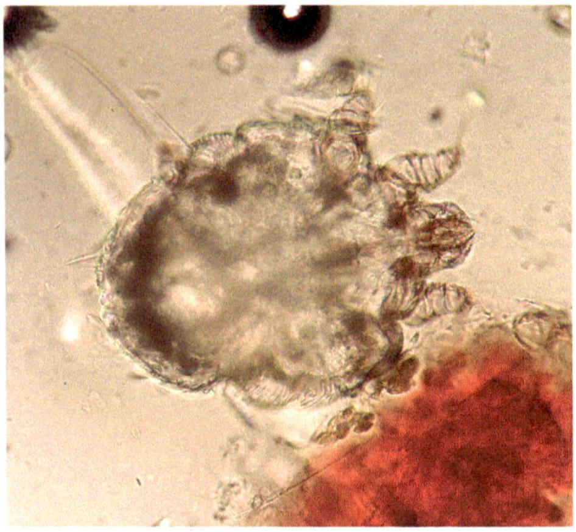

Figure 19.3. *Sarcoptes scabiei.*

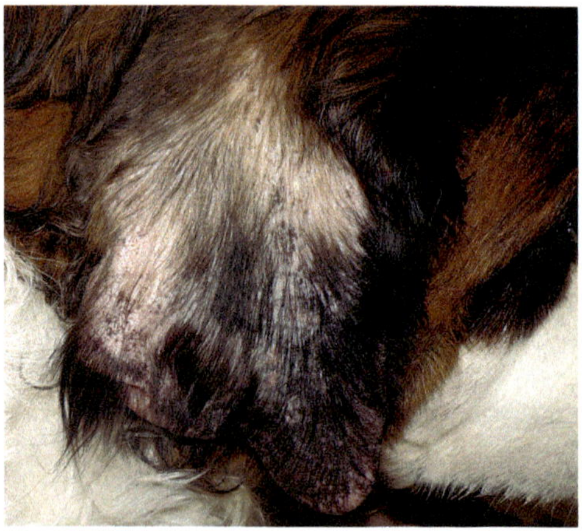

Figure 19.4. Appearance of the lesions on the pinna 3 weeks after starting acaricide treatment.

Case 20

Case presentation

The owner of a 3-year-old Maltese bitch was concerned because her dog had a pain in the flank. The dog had been spayed 15 days earlier (with no complications), but began to show signs of pain in the flank about 5 days before the consultation. On the same day the owner had discovered "strange" skin lesions. The patient ate very well and appeared not to have any other problems.

On examination of the flank the animal showed signs of pain, and clipping of the area revealed the skin lesions shown in Figure 20.1.

Questions

1. What lesions are seen in this patient?
2. What could be the cause?

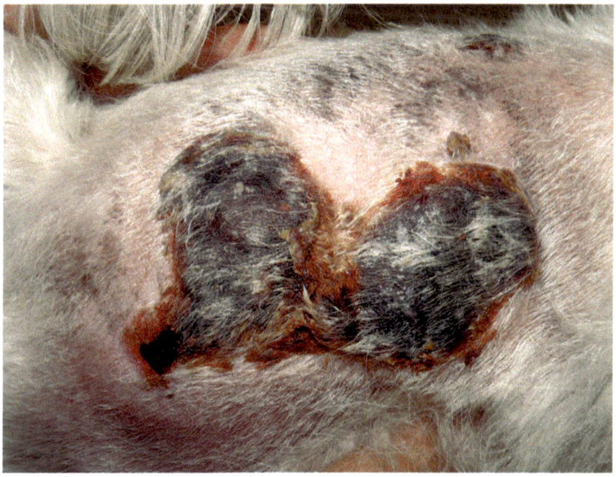

Figure 20.1. Lesions on the flank made visible after clipping.

Answers Case 20

1 What lesions are seen in this patient?

The skin lesions are very specific and indicative of cutaneous necrosis, with well-defined borders and crusting. The necrotic tissue can be clearly distinguished from the adjacent skin.

The most frequent causes of epidermal necrosis are chemical or thermal burns, vasculitis and thrombosis, traumatic vascular lesions, poisonous bites (spiders, snakes, etc.), and freezing (Fig. 20.2).

2 What could be the cause?

In the case of this animal, which had recently undergone surgery, the most likely cause of the necrosis is exposure to a heat source. Repeated and prolonged exposure to a source of moderate heat can cause a clinical lesion known by the Latin name of *erythema ab igne*. This condition is observed in dogs and cats that are exposed to heat sources such as a stoves, radiators, or electric blankets. The most commonly affected areas are the trunk and the lateral portion of the chest wall. The lesion may begin with alopecia, erythema, central depigmentation, and peripheral hyperpigmentation. It can resolve spontaneously if the heat source is removed. Otherwise, necrosis, eschar, and ulceration can occur, resulting in permanent scarring alopecia (Fig. 20.3).

In this case, the patient presented with extensive necrosis of the entire thickness of the skin, and therefore required medical treatment with antibiotics and surgical debridement of the necrotic lesions.

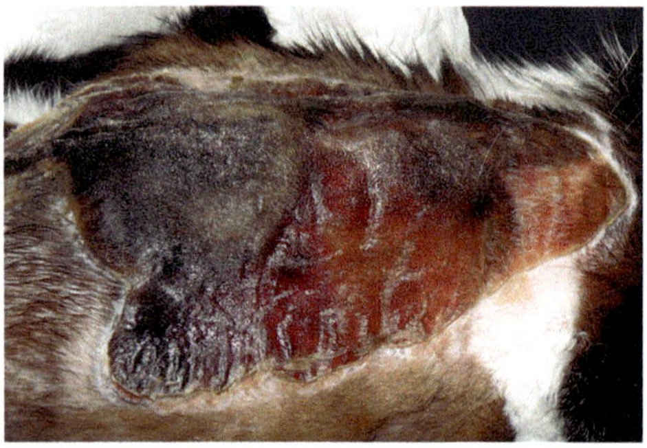

Figure 20.2. Cat with necrosis of the skin on the back secondary to prolonged contact with ice.

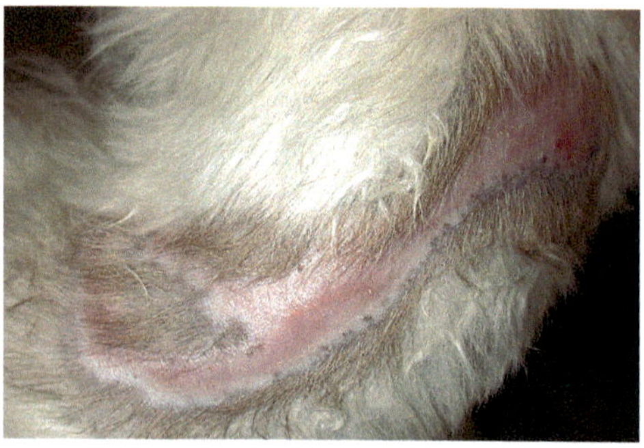

Figure 20.3. Bitch with scarring lesion caused by epidermal necrosis due to prolonged exposure to a heat source.

Case 21

Case presentation

The owner of a 1-year-old Schnauzer bitch attended the clinic with her dog, and reported noticing "little lesions" on her dog's nose. She was worried that the dog may have leishmaniasis (which another of her dogs had previously contracted). The general examination of the patient revealed no findings of note. Several lesions on the muzzle were observed (Figs. 21.1 and 21.2).

Questions

1. What lesions are observed on the muzzle?
2. What differential diagnoses should be considered based on the location of the lesions and the age of the animal?

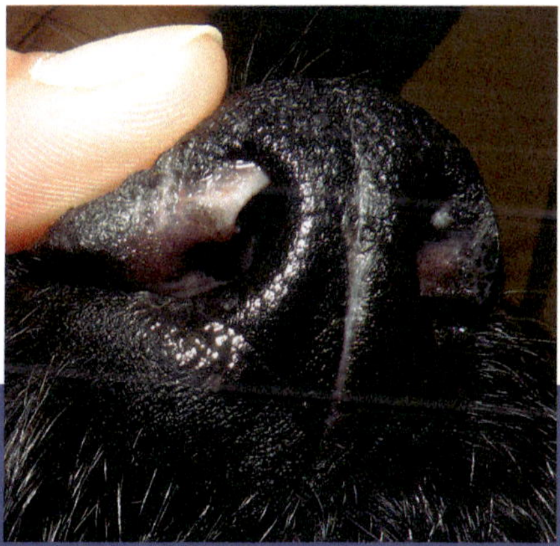

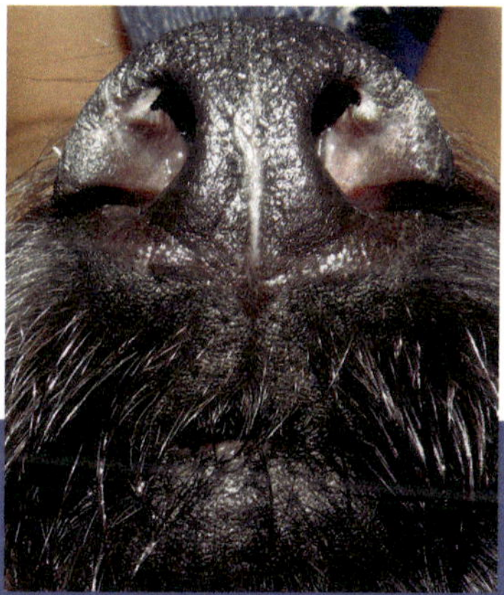

Figures 21.1 and 21.2. Appearance of the muzzle.

Answers Case 21

1 What lesions are observed on the muzzle?

The dog presented with bilateral depigmentation, mild fissures, and crusts on the muzzle and nostrils. The lesions suggest an inflammatory process. Before performing any other test, impression cytology was performed, revealing the presence of epithelial cells, neutrophils with toxic changes, and extracellular and intracellular bacteria (cocci) (Fig. 21.3).

2 What differential diagnoses should be considered based on the location of the lesions and the age of the animal?

The skin of the muzzle is specialised, and contains neither hair follicles nor glands. Given the absence of glands, the skin is hydrated by the tongue and the secretions of the nasolacrimal duct. Owing to the lack of hair, the muzzle is unaffected by follicle diseases (e.g. demodicosis), but is more sensitive to trauma and the effects of ultraviolet radiation. Diseases that produce lesions of the muzzle are usually infectious, immune-mediated, or neoplastic in nature.

In this case, given that the patient is young and healthy, and based on the cytological findings, the most likely cause of the bilateral inflammatory lesions of the muzzle would be a mucocutaneous pyoderma. However, the owner was told that if the lesions did not improve with antibiotic treatment, a histopathological study would be recommended. Serology for *Leishmania* was negative.

The lesions were treated with topical mupirocin, applied once per day. While topical treatments for the muzzle are difficult to administer, and tend not to remain on the skin for long, this antibiotic shows excellent absorption and penetration. The lesions disappeared 2 weeks after beginning topical antibiotic treatment (Fig. 21.4).

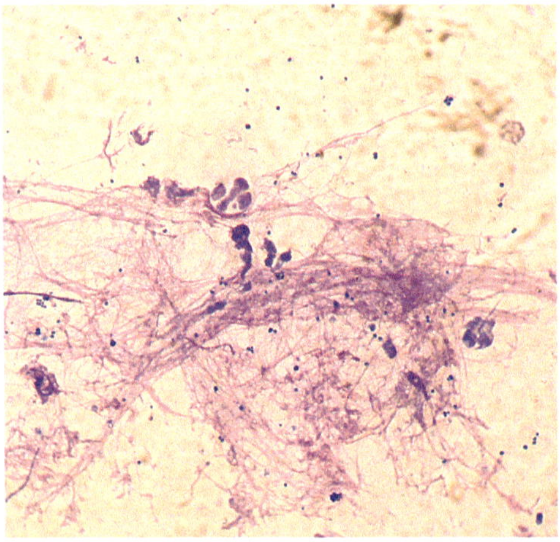

Figure 21.3. Lesion cytology showing neutrophilic granulocytes with toxic alterations and bacteria (extracellular cocci).

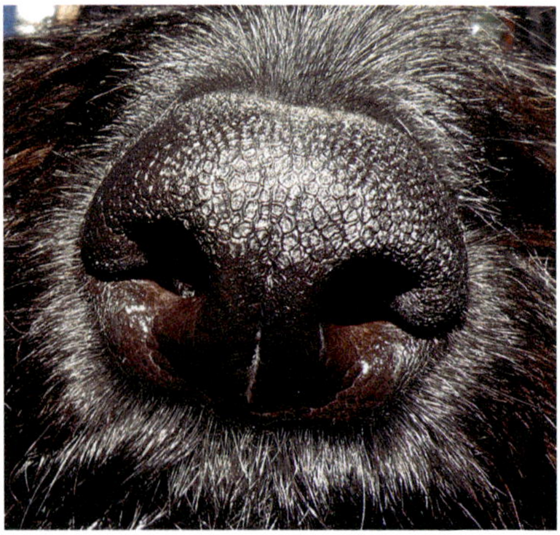

Figure 21.4. Appearance of the muzzle after treatment with antibiotics.

Case 22

Case presentation

The patient was a male dog belonging to one of our coworkers at the hospital, and had been castrated a few days earlier. The owner was very worried because her dog had developed a lesion on the skin of the scrotum that appeared to bother him (the lesion was more painful than pruritic) (Fig. 22.1).

Question

1 Could this lesion be related to the surgical procedure?

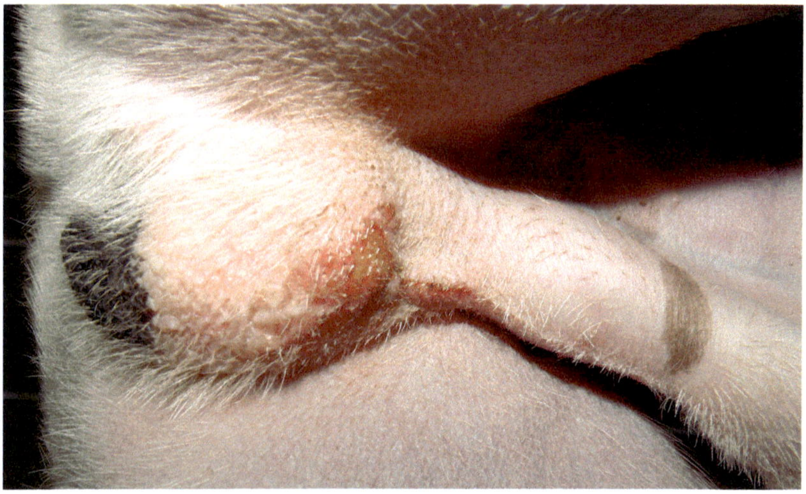

Figure 22.1. Lesion on the scrotum.

Answer Case 22

1 Could this lesion be related to the surgical procedure?

The skin lesion in question is an erosion that coincides with the area of the suture. Clipping, deep cleaning of the surgical field, and the use of antiseptic products may have caused erosion of the epidermis. In dogs the skin of the scrotum, which is less protected by the hair, may be more susceptible to contact dermatitis than other areas of the body. It is also a common site of drug reactions. The lesion resolved after a few days of treatment with topical corticosteroids.

Case 23

Case presentation

The owners of a 2-year-old castrated male fennec fox brought him to the clinic after noticing that he had been losing hair from his body and neck over the preceding 10 days. The hair loss did not appear to bother him or to cause itching, and had coincided with a period spent away from the owner's house. Three months earlier he had been treated for diarrhoea with antibiotics. His usual veterinary surgeon had performed a hair culture for dermatophytes, the results of which were negative. The patient was fed with cat food and lived in a house in the countryside with two other dogs, neither of whom had skin lesions.

The general examination revealed no findings of interest. In the dermatological examination, alopecia was detected in the trunk and the thoracolumbar area (Figs. 23.1 and 23.2). No other lesions were detected, except for an excoriation on the back that the owner attributed to playing with the dogs.

Questions

1. Does this patient have inflammatory or noninflammatory alopecia?
2. What diagnostic tests should be performed?

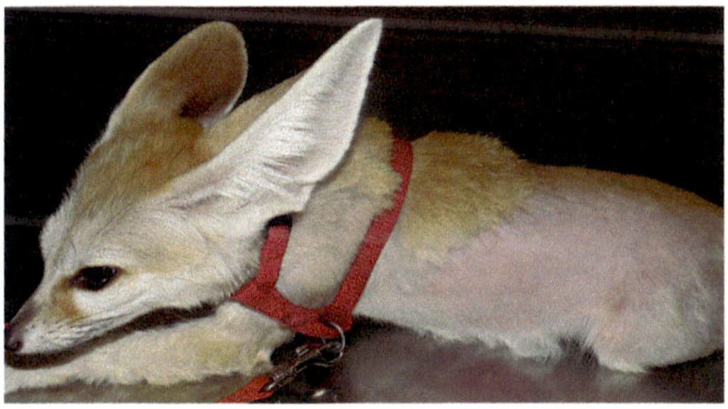

Figure 23.1. Hair loss on the trunk of the patient.

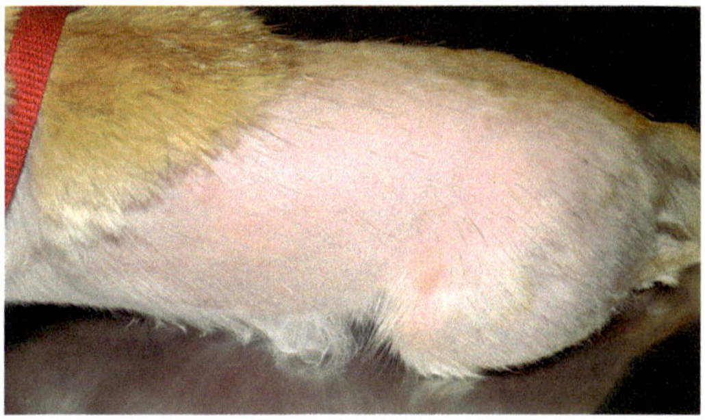

Figure 23.2. Detail of alopecia.

Answers Case 23

1 Does this patient have inflammatory or noninflammatory alopecia?

The clinical appearance is that of noninflammatory alopecia (there is no pruritus or inflammatory skin lesions), which is generalised and diffuse (not focal). The potential causes of noninflammatory and widespread alopecia in animals as young as this patient are few: congenital defects and follicular dysplasias. Genetic alopecias, such as ectodermal dysplasia, are characterised by an absence of follicles and apocrine glands, resulting in alopecia from the moment of birth. However, this fox had a normal haircoat that was suddenly lost. The animal's good general and nutritional state also appears to rule out a congenital endocrinopathy or the presence of a systemic disease.

2 What diagnostic tests should be performed?

The hair should be observed under a microscope (trichogram). In this case no parasites or infectious agents were detected, but most of the bulbs were in telogen phase (club- or spear-shaped, lacking pigmentation). The clinical signs and trichogram were compatible with telogen effluvium.

Observations

Telogen effluvium is a type of alopecia associated with stressors (high fever, gestation, shock, severe illness, surgery, medication, anaesthesia) that cause abrupt cessation of the growth of follicles in anagen phase, resulting in their synchronisation in catagen and subsequently in telogen phase. There are several forms of telogen effluvium, the most common of which occurs 3 to 5 weeks after exposure to a stressor. Diagnosis is based on the clinical history, examination results, and observation of the hair. A biopsy is rarely necessary. When alopecia due to telogen effluvium is clinically evident, histology will reveal a normal profile, with an adequate proportion of hairs in anagen phase.

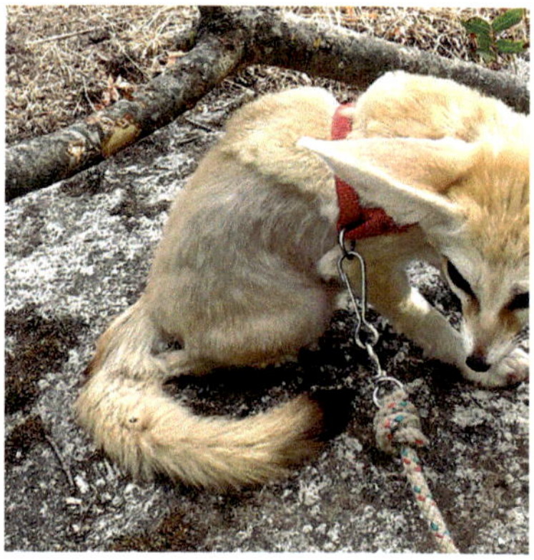

Figure 23.3. Appearance of the fennec fox 1 month after the first visit. No treatment has been administered. Hair growth is clearly evident.

Therefore, the prognosis for this patient is excellent, and he should recover his normal hair within a few weeks (Fig. 23.3).

Case 24

Case presentation

A 10-year-old mongrel dog was brought to the clinic with a small "bump" on the skin of the leg that had appeared 1 month previously. The owner had noticed that the nodule had grown slightly during the preceding week. The general condition of the dog was good. On examination, a firm, ulcerated skin nodule was observed on the skin of the plantar surface of the fourth digit of the right hindlimb (Figs. 24.1 and 24.2). Fine-needle aspiration cytology of the nodule was performed (Figs. 24.3 and 24.4).

Questions

1 What is the most likely diagnosis based on the clinical appearance of the lesion and the cytological findings?

2 What are the treatment of choice and prognosis for this pathology?

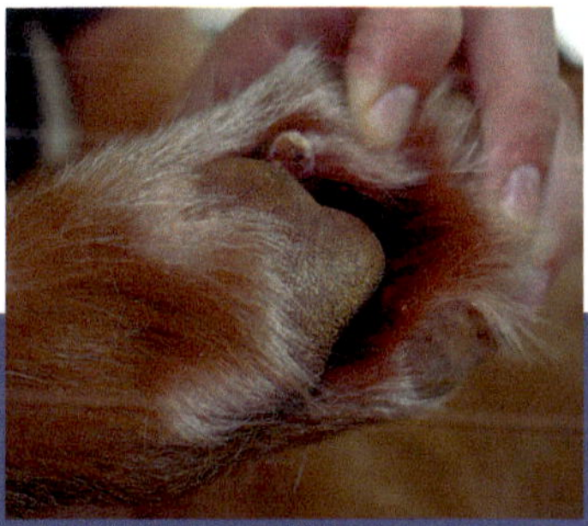

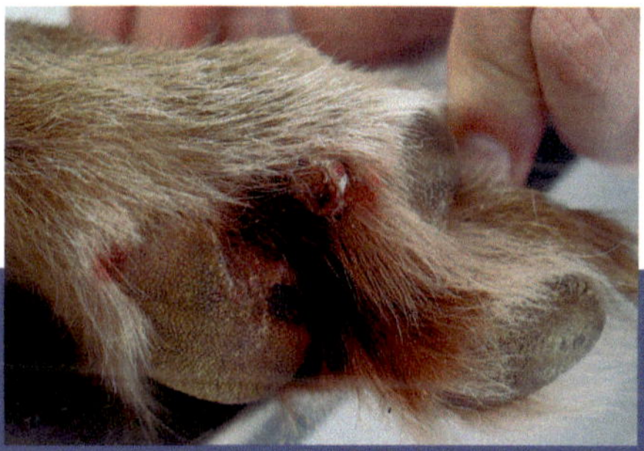

Figures 24.1 and 24.2. Firm, ulcerated skin nodule on the skin of the fourth digit.

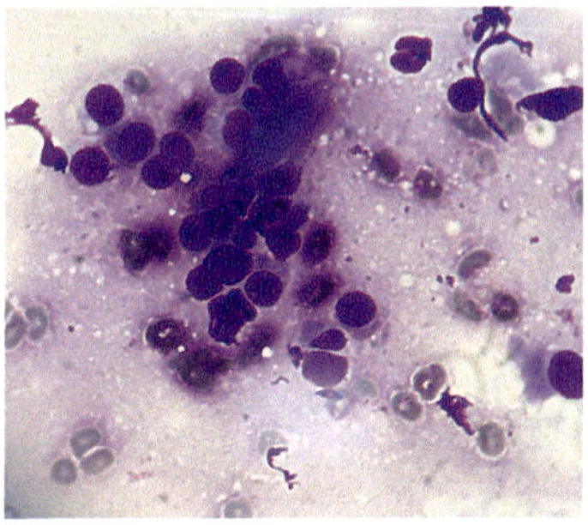

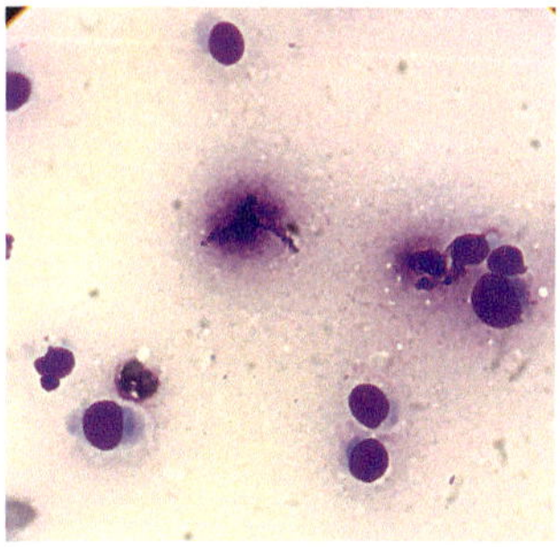

Figures 24.3 and 24.4. Fine-needle aspiration cytology of the nodule.

Answers Case 24

1 What is the most likely diagnosis based on the clinical appearance of the lesion and the cytological findings?

Cytology showed small, well-differentiated cells, with a round or oval appearance, an eccentric nucleus, regular chromatin, and cytoplasm with clear areas behind the nucleus (Golgi apparatus). Some binucleated cells were evident. This cytological profile is highly suggestive of a plasmacytoma.

Cutaneous plasmacytoma is a neoplasm that originates in plasma cells. It is rare in dogs, with a higher incidence in older dogs. It manifests as multiple solitary, well-defined, white, firm skin nodules, which can be pedunculated or ulcerated and erythematous, and which vary in size from a few millimetres to several centimetres in diameter. These lesions are most commonly found on the lips, digits, limbs, pinnae, and the nose (Fig. 24.5).

2 What are the treatment of choice and prognosis for this pathology?

Surgical excision is the treatment of choice. The prognosis is good in dogs, and local recurrence and metastasis are unlikely.

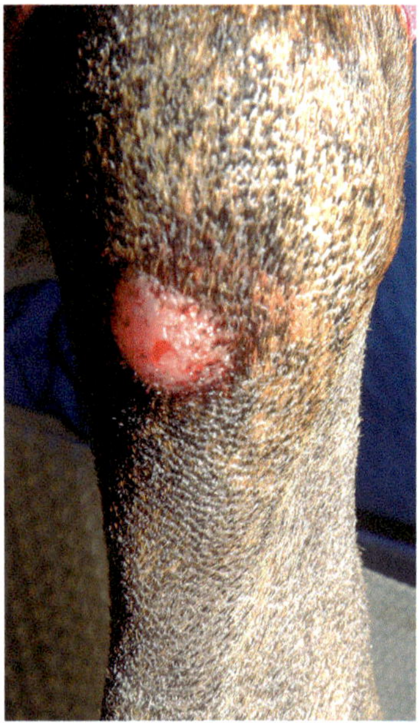

Figure 24.5. Cutaneous plasmacytoma on the limb of a dog.

Case 25

Case presentation

The owners of a male Russian Blue cat attended the dermatology department with their pet, who had lesions on the ears and eyelids that had appeared 3 years earlier. Some lumps appeared in the summer and disappeared in October. The lesions caused significant itching. The cat did not live with other animals and the owners had no skin lesions. They lived in an apartment in the capital, but travelled frequently to another city. The cat had received antiparasitic treatment for internal parasites only.

The general examination revealed no findings of note, except for slight overweight. Crusted papular lesions were observed on the pinna and the preauricular area (Figs. 25.1 and 25.2). No lesions were detected anywhere else on the body.

Lesion cytology showed numerous neutrophilic and eosinophilic granulocytes.

Questions

1. What is the most likely cause of this clinical picture?
2. What is the appropriate treatment?

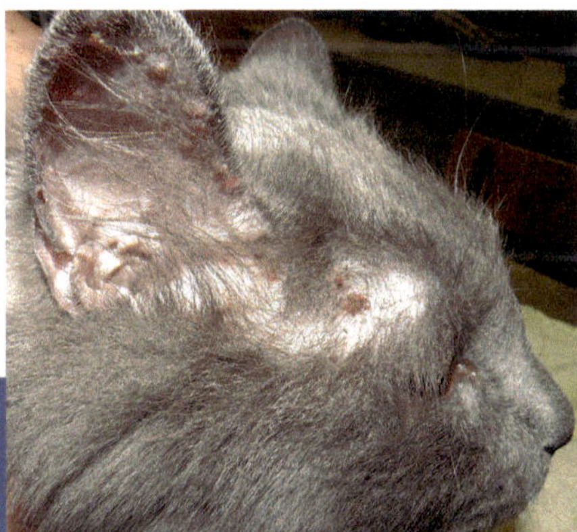

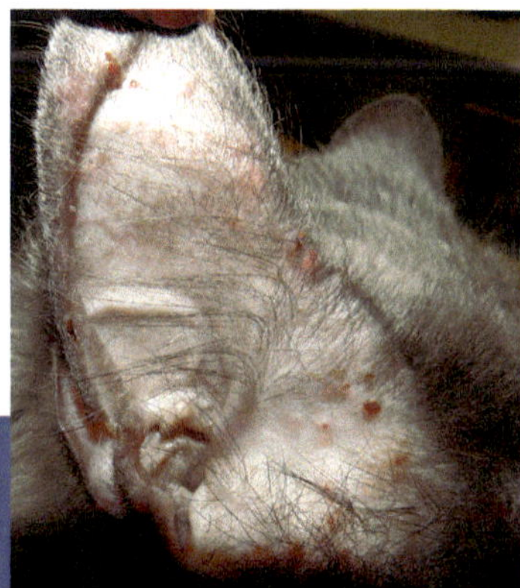

Figures 25.1 and 25.2. Crusted papular lesions on the pinna and in the preauricular area.

Answers Case 25

1 What is the most likely cause of this clinical picture?

The clinical signs suggest hypersensitivity to mosquito bites, although other differential diagnoses should be taken into account, including other types of allergies, dermatophytosis, otoacariasis, demodicosis, and pemphigus foliaceus.

Hypersensitivity to mosquito bites is a rare seasonal disease that is observed in cats that are sensitised to the bites of these insects.

Crusted papules or pustules appear on the bridge of the nose and on the outside part of the ears. The outer edges of the footpads can also be affected, with hyperkeratosis, hyperpigmentation, and fissures, which can be very painful.

2 What is the appropriate treatment?

Treatment consists of confining the cat in a mosquito-free environment, especially at dawn and dusk. Lesions can be treated with prednisolone until resolution. Pyrethroid products should not be used to treat cats as they can be toxic. However, insecticide for environmental diffusion can be used.

Case 26

Case presentation

A spayed female Breton Spaniel of 10 years of age was referred by a fellow veterinary surgeon with chronic lesions on the nose. The lesions had appeared 1 year earlier. She was being treated with prednisolone at low doses, but the lesions had worsened and spread to the leg. She had also been treated with a menthol-based topical product. The dog had significant pruritus and was very dejected. Poor body condition and moderate lymphadenopathy were observed in the general examination.

The dermatological examination revealed a severe facial condition with highly exudative, crusted, and ulcerative lesions that affected the entire nasal bridge, eyelids, and dermoepidermal junction, but not the muzzle. The dog also had hyperkeratosis and fissures of the plantar pads, as well as exudative and crusted lesions on the distal portion of the limbs, with nail dystrophy (Figs. 26.1–26.3).

The results of the superficial and deep scrapings and the Wood's lamp examination were all negative. Cytology showed a pyogranulomatous exudate with low numbers of intracellular microorganisms (cocci) and the presence of eosinophils, mast cells, and small amounts of plasma cells.

Questions

1. What pathologies should be included in the differential diagnosis of this clinical picture?
2. What diagnostic tests should be performed?

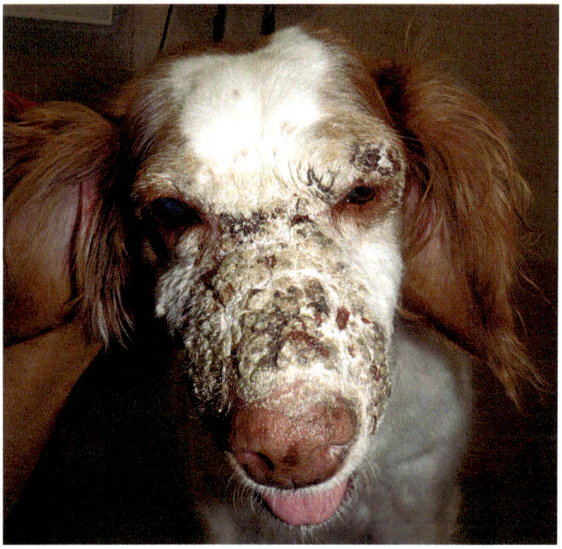

Figure 26.1. Severe crusted lesions on the nasal bridge, eyelids, and dermoepidermal junction.

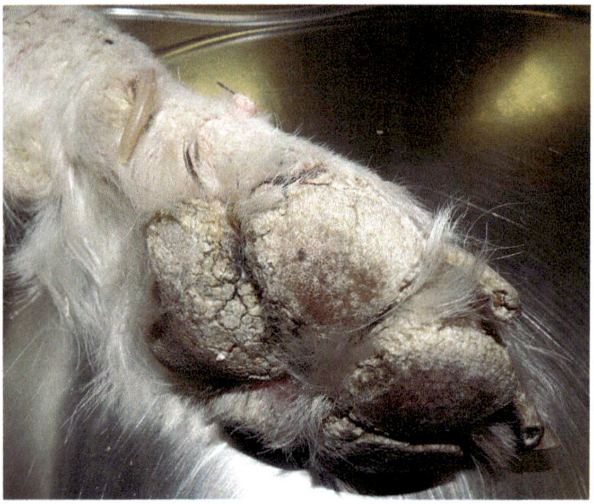

Figure 26.2. Hyperkeratosis and fissures on the footpads.

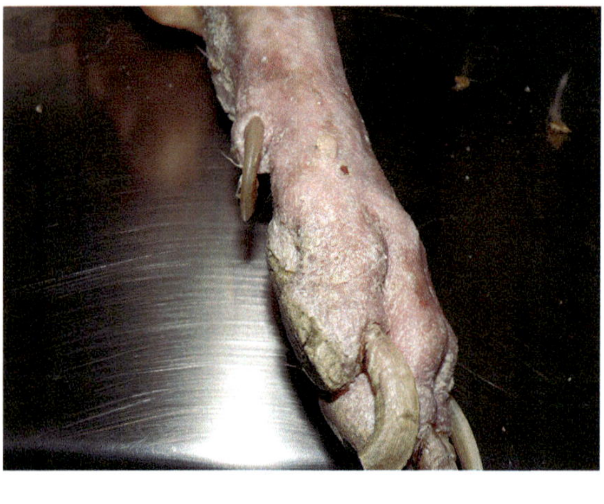

Figure 26.3. Nail dystrophy

Answers Case 26

1 What pathologies should be included in the differential diagnosis of this clinical picture?

The following are the most likely differential diagnoses for these clinical signs:

- Pemphigus foliaceus.
- Leishmaniasis.
- Deep pyoderma complicated with atypical or multiresistant bacteria.
- Drug reaction.

2 What diagnostic tests should be performed?

In this case, blood tests and serology for infectious diseases (leishmaniasis and canine ehrlichiosis) were performed, the results of which were negative. Bacterial culture revealed the presence of *Staphylococcus pseudintermedius*, which was sensitive to beta-lactam antibiotics. However, the patient showed only a partial response to oral cephalexin treatment. Histopathology showed epithelial hyperplasia with marked hyperkeratosis and the presence of arthroconidia in the superficial keratin and in the infundibulum in some follicles (Fig. 26.4). Culture in DTM medium was positive for colonies of *Trichophyton mentagrophytes*. The dog was treated with oral ketoconazole, with a good response (Fig. 26.5).

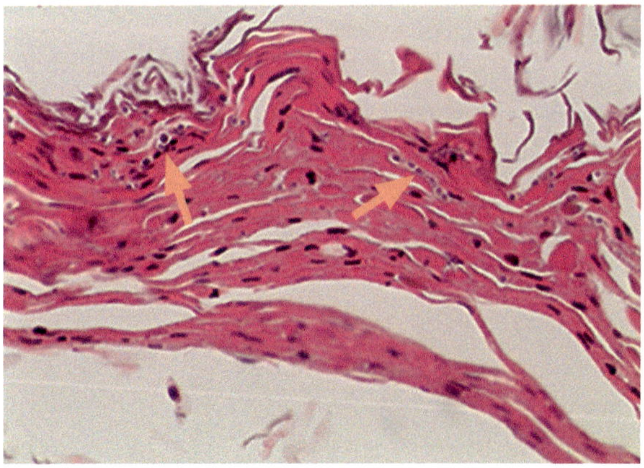

Figure 26.4. Histological image in which hyphae are observed in the stratum corneum (arrows).

Observations

Superficial pustular dermatophytosis is a rare skin disorder. It is caused by dermatophytes that colonise the surface of the stratum corneum. *Trichophyton mentagrophytes* var. *erinacei* is the most common causative keratinophilic agent, the natural reservoir of which is the European hedgehog.

This syndrome has a different presentation to most cases of dermatophytosis and can resemble an autoimmune process both clinically and histologically (acantholysis). It has been proposed that acantholysis may be the result of an immune-mediated reaction involving the release of proteolytic enzymes. Furthermore, this type of dermatophyte is not as well adapted to the host and induces a more pronounced cellular response.

The lesions consist of pustular formations that quickly rupture causing crusting, erosion, and ulceration. The most commonly affected location is the face, including the muzzle, the nasal bridge, and the periorbital region.

Unlike other dermatophyte infections, the nasal plane and footpads can be affected, and the distribution can be symmetrical.

Superficial pustular dermatophytosis has been linked to states of immunosuppression.

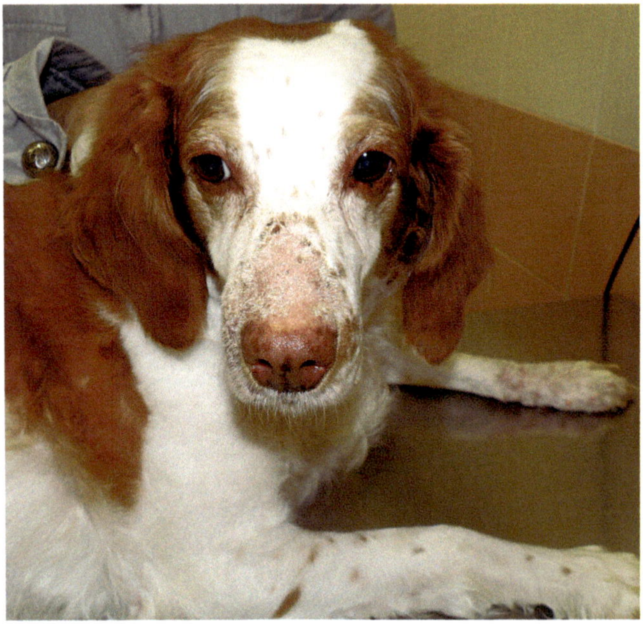

Figure 26.5. Appearance of the patient after 2 weeks of treatment with oral ketoconazole.

Case 27

Case presentation

A female Maine Coon cat of 2 years of age presented with facial pruritus that had appeared 1 month earlier. Onset coincided with a stay of 1 month in a small town in the countryside, where the cat and her brother had spent time outdoors. The cat was vaccinated during the first year of life, but had not been revaccinated since. She had received no antiparasitic treatment for either external or internal parasites. The other cat had no lesions.

The general examination revealed poor body condition, but no other findings of note. In the dermatological examination, crusted papules and excoriations were observed in the preauricular area and on the neck (Fig. 27.1). Results of basic tests (scraping, brushing, and trichogram) were normal. Lesion cytology showed eosinophils and neutrophils with intracellular microorganisms (cocci). A dermatophyte culture was performed and the patient received symptomatic treatment with amoxicillin/clavulanic acid (20 mg/kg PO every 12 hours), prednisolone (2 mg/kg/day PO), and topical selamectin (pipette).

In follow-up 10 days later, the cat showed signs of hyporexia, continued weight loss, and facial pruritus. New lesions had also developed. There were fissures and hyperkeratosis on the footpads, and an exudate around the nails, which were fragmented (Figs. 27.2 and 27.3). Exudate was also observed around the nipples. Dermatophyte culture had been negative up to this point. Given the poor response to symptomatic treatment and the presence of systemic clinical signs, a blood test was performed, revealing neutropaenia, anaemia, and severe thrombocytopaenia.

Questions

1. What is the most likely cause of severe pancytopaenia in young cats?
2. Could this be related to the dermatological signs?

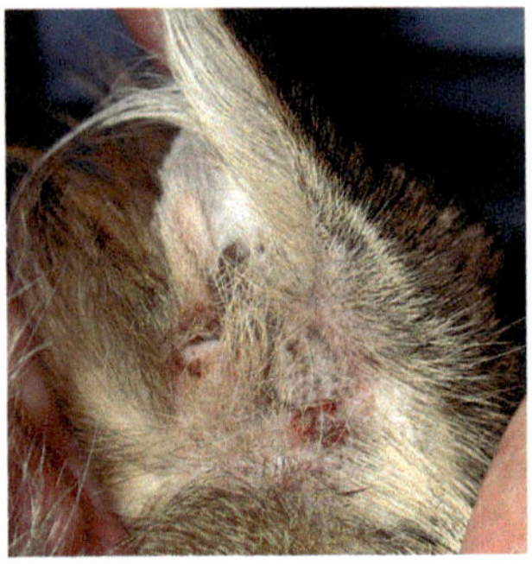

Figure 27.1. Erythema and crusted papular lesions in the preauricular area.

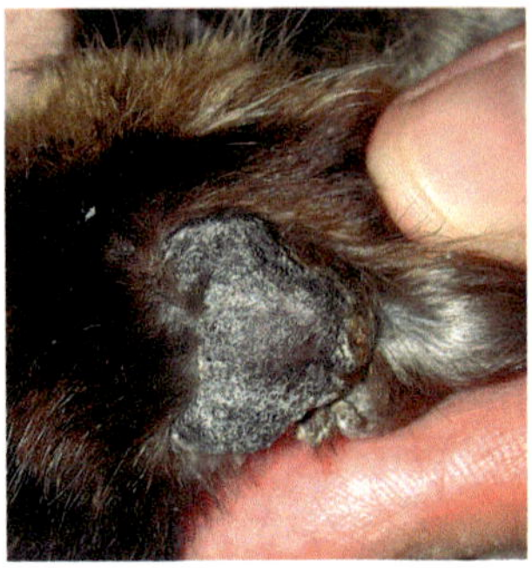

Figure 27.2. Hyperkeratosis, crusts, and scaling of the footpads.

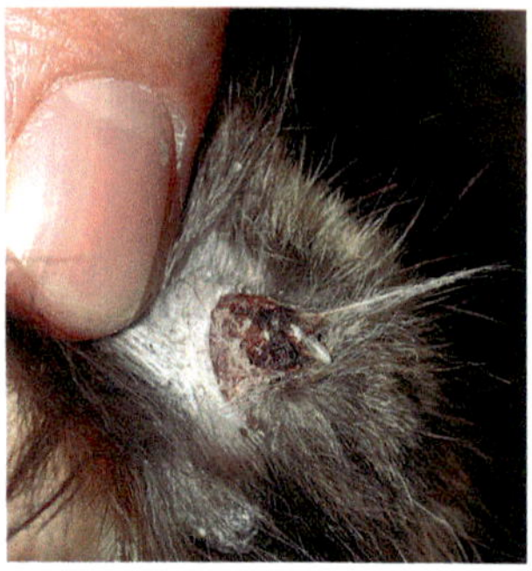

Figure 27.3. Haemorrhagic exudate around the nail.

Answers Case 27

1 What is the most likely cause of severe pancytopaenia in young cats?

Retrovirus infection is the most frequent cause of pancytopaenia in young cats. In this clinical case, the cat was positive for feline leukaemia virus.

2 Could this be related to the dermatological signs?

Several cutaneous diseases associated with feline leukaemia virus have been described. Giant cell dermatosis is a disease characterised by scaling and pruritus involving the face, digits, footpads, and mammary gland region. It owes its name to the formation of giant syncytial cells (altered keratinocytes). Other skin diseases associated with feline leukaemia virus are a result of the immunosuppression induced by this viral infection. Feline leukaemia virus has also been associated with the appearance of cutaneous horns and an increased incidence of cutaneous lymphoma.

The owners of the cat declined to consent to a biopsy to confirm the diagnosis. Given the poor response to symptomatic treatment, they decided to euthanise the animal.

Despite its low incidence, feline leukaemia virus infection should be included in the differential diagnosis of pruritic facial dermatoses of cats.

Case 28

Case presentation

The owner of a cattery breeding Norwegian Forest cats came to our centre with several animals that had developed skin lesions 1 week earlier. One of the cats, a 3-year-old female, had highly pruritic erythematous plaques on the head and neck (Fig. 28.1). Another, a 2-year-old male, exhibited crusted papules in the thoracolumbar region. A third, 6-month-old cat had symmetrical hypotrichosis in the lateral trunk area (Fig. 28.2). The general condition of all three cats was good and they had not been outdoors, except for the female who had participated in a cat competition several weeks earlier.

Basic dermatological tests (examination of hair and scales after brushing and a skin scraping) were negative for all three animals. Hair culture in DTM medium, performed to rule out dermatophytosis, was negative in all cases.

The owner was informed that flea bite was the most likely cause of the skin lesions, and the cats were treated with fipronil (pipette). The animals with miliary dermatitis and alopecia improved slightly over the following few days. However, in the female the pruritus persisted, and new lesions appeared.

Ten days later, a 2-month-old kitten from the same cattery was brought to the clinic with severe pruritus, dorsal scaling, and hypotrichosis. Examination of the hair and scaling revealed the presence of a parasite (Fig. 28.3). This kitten had never been outdoors and had only been in contact with the other cats in the cattery.

Questions

1. What parasite is this?
2. What is the best method for microscopic observation of this parasite?
3. Could it account for the clinical signs observed in the other cats?

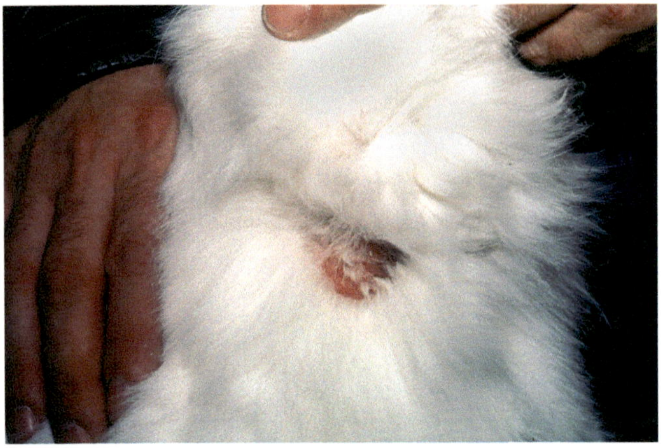

Figure 28.1. Erythema, exudation, and excoriation of the skin of the neck.

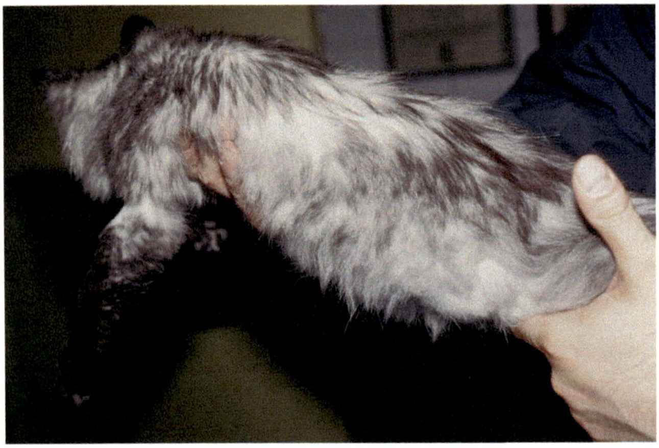

Figure 28.2. Hypotrichosis on the side of the trunk.

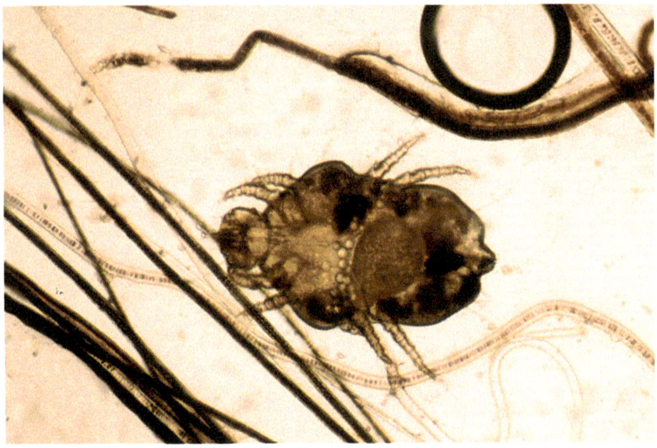

Figure 28.3. Mite detected after microscopic examination of brushed hair.

Answers Case 28

1 What parasite is this?

This is a mite of the species *Cheyletiella blakei.* Cheyletiellosis is a acariosis that is often underdiagnosed in cats. *Cheyletiella* mites live on the surface of the skin and feed on skin debris. The external environment, in which the parasites can survive for at least a month, plays an important role in contagion. Cheyletiellosis mainly affects young cats (less than 1 year old), although adults can be asymptomatic carriers. In some breeds, especially those with long hair, it is an enzootic disease that causes high morbidity. Contagion of humans is reported in 20–30 % of cat infections. Human infection is characterised by pruritus and crusted papular lesions on the arms and trunk. Once the animal has been cured, the lesions on humans disappear spontaneously within 3 weeks.

2 What is the best method for microscopic observation of this parasite?

Cats with pruritus are particularly adept at eliminating evidence of external parasites of the skin surface and hair, and therefore microscopic examination of skin scrapings or samples obtained with adhesive tape produce negative results. Of the techniques mentioned, the one preferred by many authors is microscopic examination of scales and hair obtained by brushing, since the eggs of the parasite adhere to the surface of the hair and remain attached to the skin for longer than other stages of the life cycle of *Cheyletiella.* However, examination after brushing can be negative in 58 % of cats. Another diagnostic technique is faecal flotation, which may reveal the presence of mites and eggs ingested by the cat by licking.

3 Could it account for the clinical signs observed in the other cats?

Although the classical clinical picture in dogs and cats is a keratoseborrhoeic disorder (Fig. 28.4), the clinical signs of parasitisation by *Cheyletiella* resemble those of other inflammatory and pruritic processes in cats, and can manifest clinically as any of the four classic patterns of pruritus seen in cats: self-induced alopecia, miliary dermatitis, eosinophilic granuloma complex, and facial pruritus. In some animals, such as the adult female cat described in this clinical case, the intensity of pruritus is not directly related to the number of parasites, suggesting potential hypersensitivity to the mite.

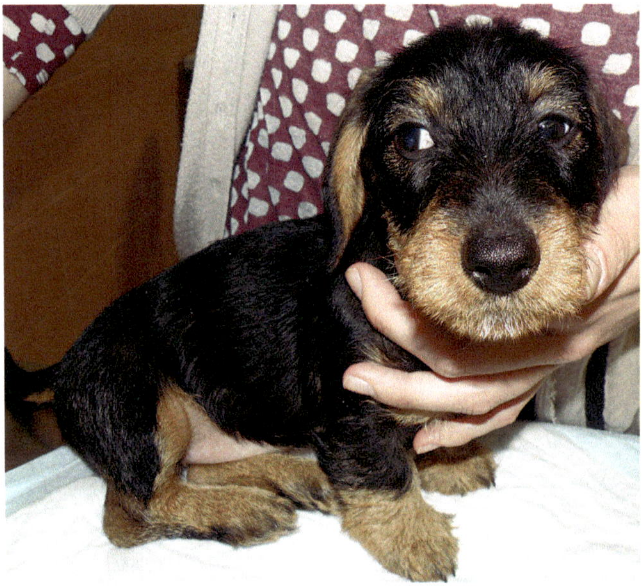

Figure 28.4. Keratoseborrhoeic disorder in a puppy with cheyletiellosis.

Case 29

Case presentation

The owner of a male cryptorchid American Pitbull Terrier, aged 4 years, attended the veterinary clinic and reported that his dog appeared to have lost hair from the lower back. The dog had been adopted at 6 months of age and was the smallest of his litter. At the time of the consultation, pruritus was absent and the dog's general condition was good. Examination revealed hypotrichosis in the dorsal area (Figs. 29.1 and 29.2), but no other skin lesions. A trichogram was performed (Fig. 29.3).

Questions

1. What is observed in the trichogram?
2. What is this patient's diagnosis?

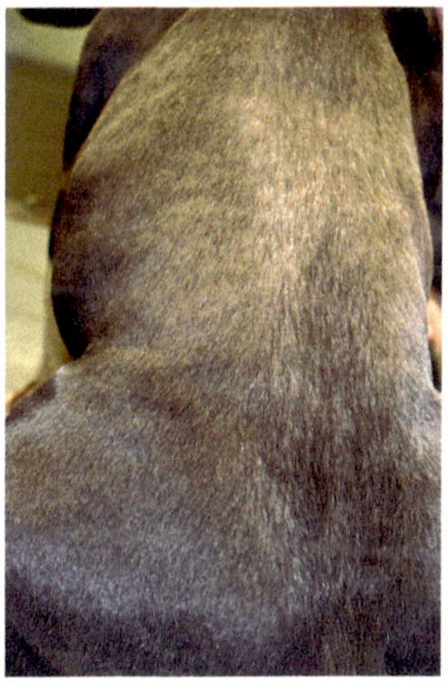

Figure 29.1. Hypotrichosis and diffuse alopecia in the dorsal part of the trunk.

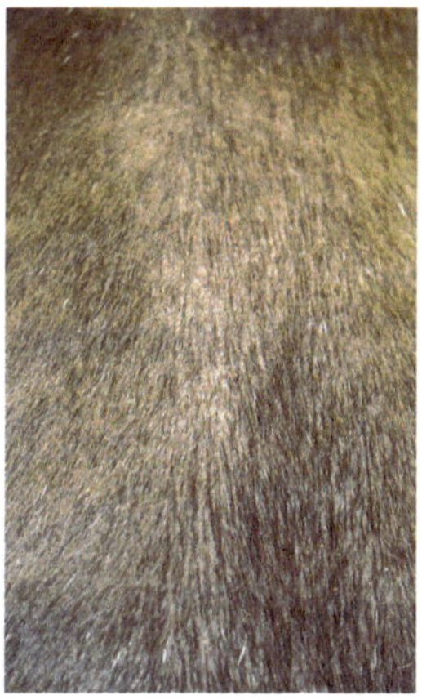

Figure 29.2. Detail of the alopecic area.

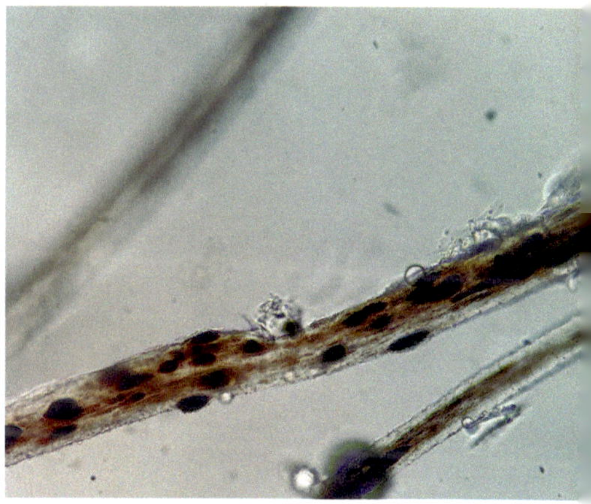

Figure 29.3. Trichogram of the same dog.

Answers Case 29

1 What is observed in the trichogram?

Large melanin granules (macromelanosomes) are evident in the trichogram. These granules can become grouped, giving rise to areas of fragility and resulting in secondary rupture of the diaphysis, and consequent hypotrichosis or alopecia (Fig. 29.4).

2 What is this patient's diagnosis?

This pathology is observed in dogs with a diluted haircoat and is a type of follicular dysplasia with a hereditary component. It is common in dogs with a diluted haircoat (grey or blue and beige). Affected dogs appear normal when they are born, but begin to lose hair from the dorsal trunk area between 6 months and 2 years of age. Only diluted hairs are lost, and secondary superficial pyoderma may be observed.

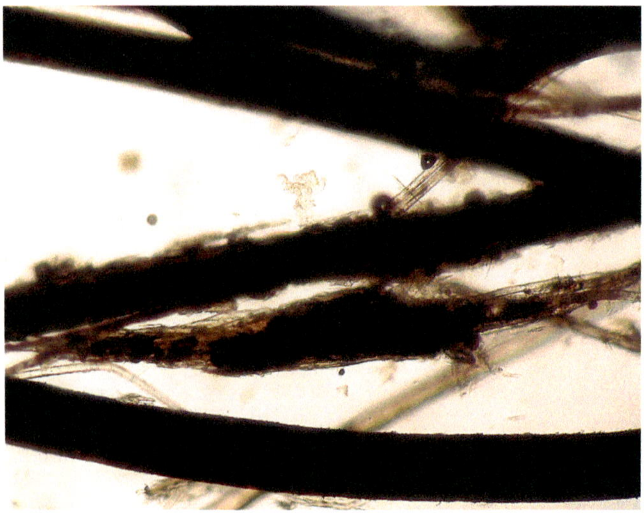

Figure 29.4. Macromelanosome that is about to cause breakage of the diaphysis of the hair.

Case 30

Case presentation

The patient, a 2-year-old male Golden Retriever, presented with generalised scaling that had begun 2 months earlier. Pruritus was absent and the dog's general condition was good. Abundant greyish scaling was observed in the dermatological examination (Figs. 30.1–30.3). There were no clinical signs indicative of inflammation or alopecia, or of the presence of parasites or infectious agents. Keratin remnants were visible in the scales when viewed under the microscope (Fig. 30.4).

Questions

1. What type of dermatological disorder does this dog have?
2. What could have caused it?

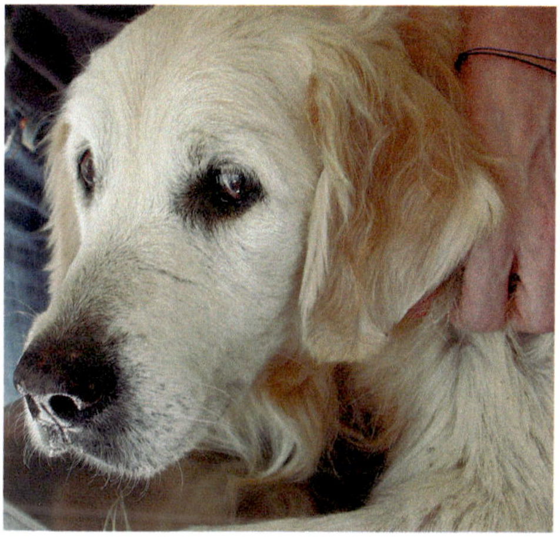

Figure 30.1. Golden Retriever patient with greyish scaling. ▶

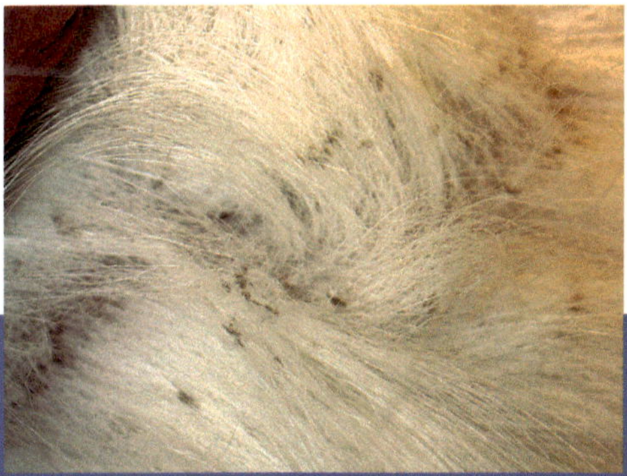

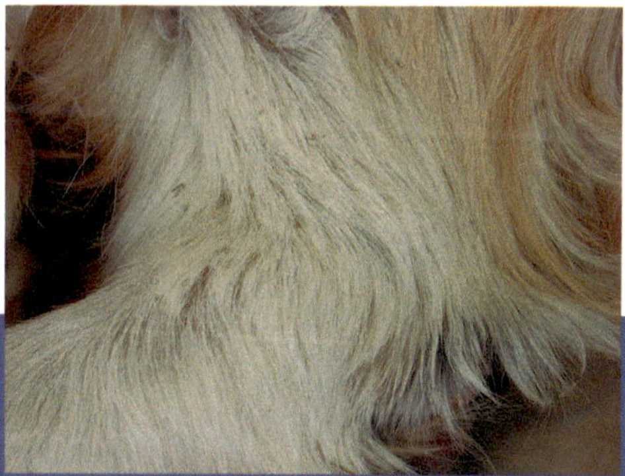

Figures 30.2 and 30.3. Detail of the scaling on the trunk and limbs.

Answers Case 30

1 What type of dermatological disorder does this dog have?

The dog has a keratoseborrhoeic condition.

2 What could have caused it?

The majority of seborrhoeic disorders in dogs are secondary to inflammatory or endocrine processes. However, in this case, given the absence of other clinical signs, it appears to be a primary disorder. The breed and the type of scaling suggest laminar ichthyosis.

Ichthyosis is a congenital disease that affects the stratum corneum and is present from the moment of birth, although it may not be very noticeable and can worsen over time. It is characterised by scaling, whereby skin detaches in large sheets or accumulates in flakes on the surface of the skin. Lesions may appear on the nose and footpads, with intense hyperkeratosis.

Histology shows orthokeratotic hyperkeratosis, with accumulations of keratin at the entrance of the follicular infundibulum (Fig. 30.5).

Treatment is symptomatic, and improvement may be observed with the use of antiseborrhoeic and emollient shampoos, although this is a chronic and incurable disorder.

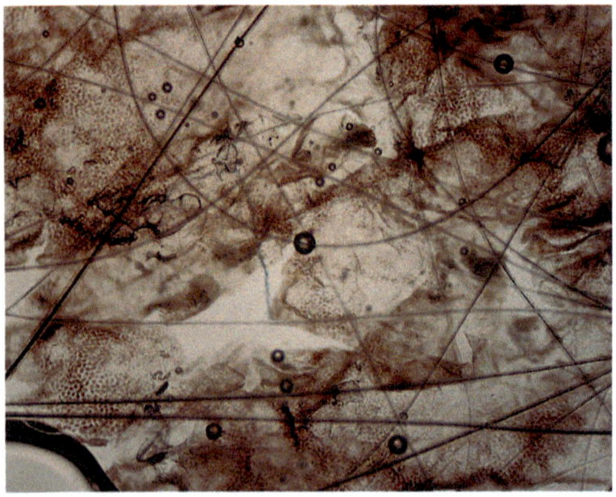

Figure 30.4. Appearance of scaling under the microscope.

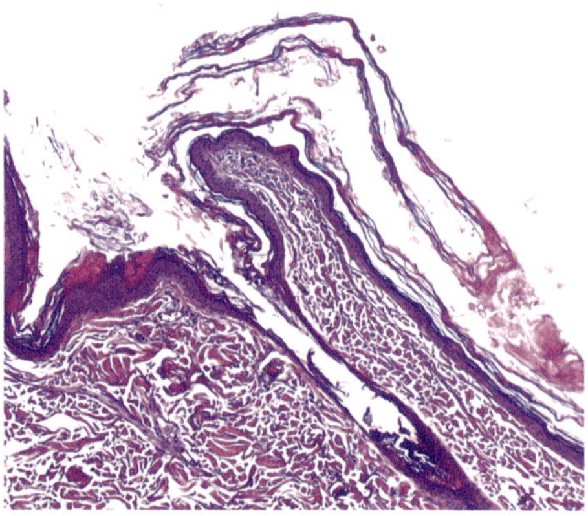

Figure 30.5. Histological image showing orthokeratotic hyperkeratosis.

Case 31

Case presentation

A 2-year-old male mongrel dog arrived at the hospital for surgery on a torn anterior cruciate ligament. The owner reported that he had observed a lump on the skin of one of the forelimbs several weeks earlier (Fig. 31.1). A single alopecic, erythematous nodular lesion with a firm appearance was observed (Fig. 31.2). Fine-needle aspiration cytology was performed (Figs. 31.3–31.5).

Questions

1 What pathologies should be included in the differential diagnosis of this type of lesion in a young dog?

2 What does the lesion cytology show and what is the most likely diagnosis?

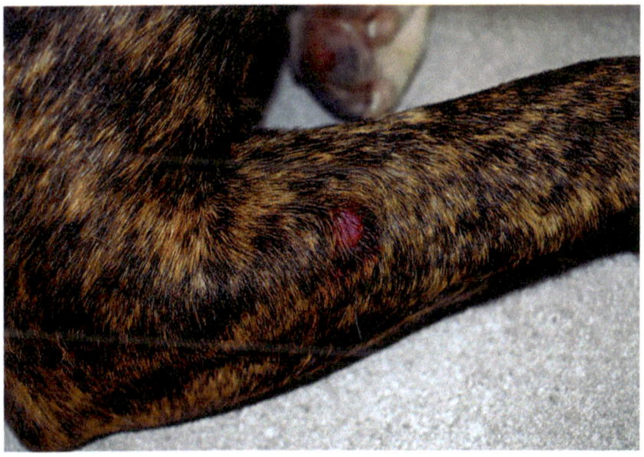

Figure 31.1. Patient's skin nodule.

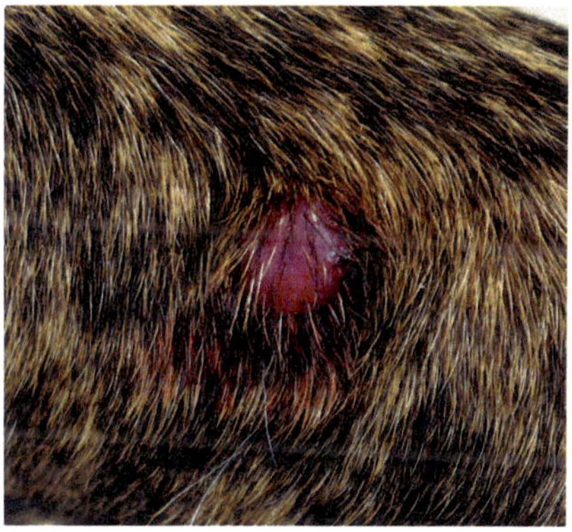

Figure 31.2. Appearance of the alopecic and erythematous nodule.

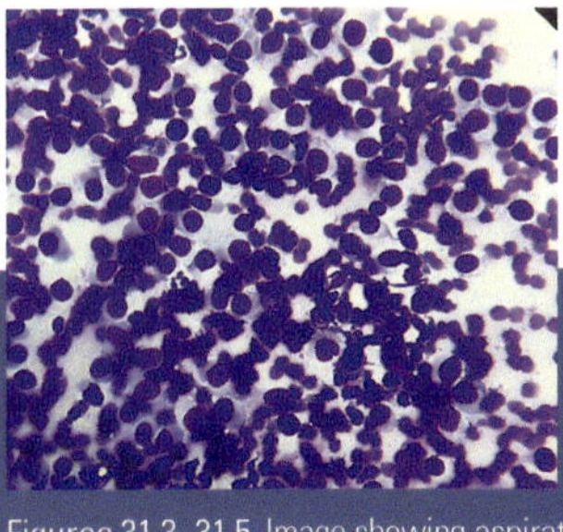

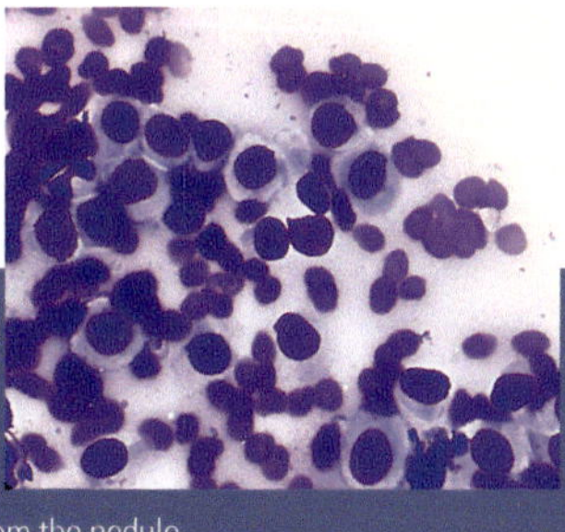

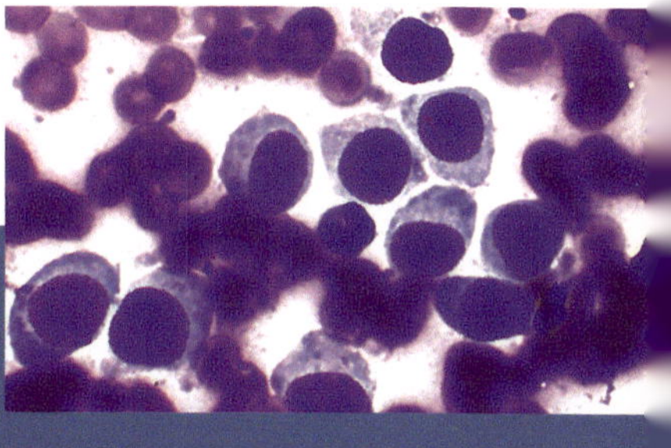

Figures 31.3–31.5. Image showing aspirate from the nodule.

Answers Case 31

1 What pathologies should be included in the differential diagnosis of this type of lesion in a young dog?

The differential diagnosis of a cutaneous nodular lesion in a young dog should include:

- Pyogranulomatous inflammatory processes.
- Dermatophyte kerion.
- Nodular leishmaniasis.
- Cutaneous histiocytoma.

2 What does the lesion cytology show and what is the most likely diagnosis?

Cytology shows numerous large round cells, with a moderate amount of light blue, finely granulated cytoplasm. The nucleus is round or kidney-shaped, with fine chromatin. The cytological profile corresponds to a cutaneous histiocytoma.

Observations

Histiocytomas are benign tumours of the skin that originate in epithelial Langerhans cells. In general, they appear as solitary lesions, which usually disappear spontaneously. Multiple histiocytomas only occur in 1 % of cases and are more common in Shar Peis. Although they are very rare, recurrence and metastasis of this type of tumour have been described.

Histiocytomas are progressively invaded by lymphocytes and enter remission over a variable period of time (Fig. 31.6). Neoplastic histiocytes undergo lysis caused by the cytotoxic effects of infiltrating lymphocytes. Observation without treatment is a reasonable protocol, since most lesions resolve spontaneously in less than 3 months. Surgical excision or cryotherapy are curative for lesions that do not remit spontaneously.

The prognosis for this type of benign tumour is good.

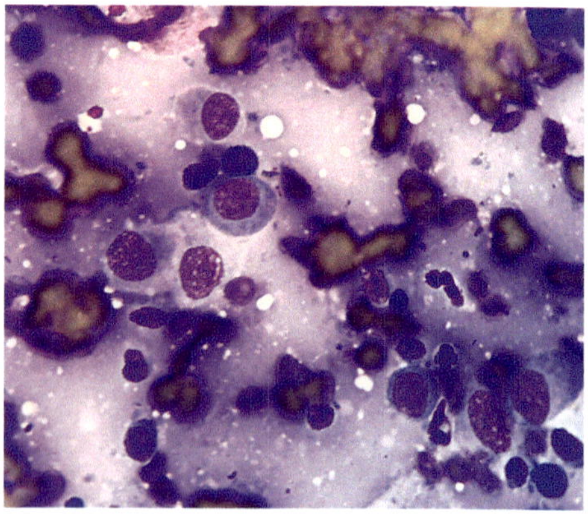

Figure 31.6. Cytological image of a cutaneous histiocytoma in regression; mature lymphocytes as well as characteristic histiocytic cells are observed.

Case 32

Case presentation

The patient was an intact, male mongrel dog, aged 7 years, with small hairless patches that had developed on the back of his neck. He appeared unperturbed by the lesions. The dog had been hospitalised 4 weeks earlier for a cervical vertebral problem. Localised areas of alopecia were observed in the general examination (Figs. 32.1 and 32.2).

Questions

1. Is this dog's alopecia inflammatory or noninflammatory?
2. What is the most likely cause?

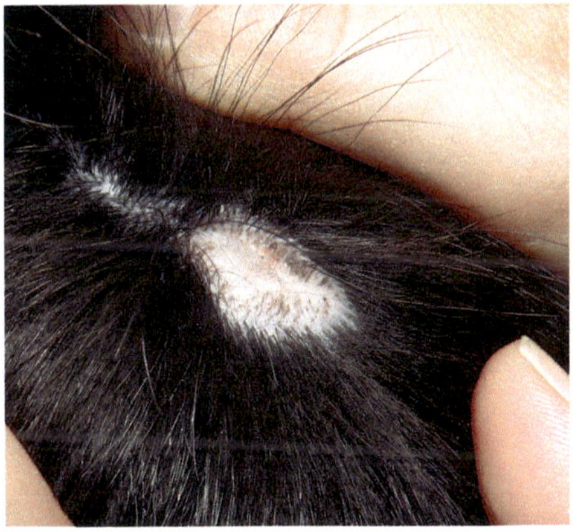

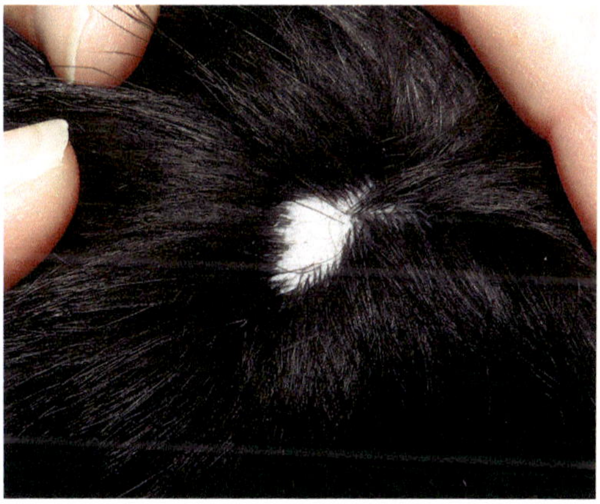

Figures 32.1 and 32.2. Focal alopecia in the neck area.

Answers Case 32

1 Is this dog's alopecia inflammatory or noninflammatory?

The alopecia affecting this dog appears to be noninflammatory, since inflammatory clinical signs (e.g. erythema, pruritus) are absent. The skin appears atrophic and hypopigmented. However, histopathology of the lesions could reveal mild inflammatory infiltrate.

2 What is the most likely cause?

Post-injection alopecia is the most likely cause of these multifocal hairless areas. Alopecia secondary to injection is the result of panniculitis followed by a subsequent ischaemic reaction, which in turn causes alopecia and cutaneous atrophy. It is associated with the injection of corticosteroids, vaccines, and progestogens, but can also be caused by other medications.

A focal, circumscribed oval or circular area of alopecia forms at the injection site. Erythema and scaling may be observed initially. The skin has a thin, atrophic, and hyper- or hypopigmented appearance. Lesions can appear between 1 and 4 months after the injection. In vaccine-associated alopecia, multifocal alopecia caused by vasculitis may be observed around the primary lesion (Figs. 32.3 and 32.4). These secondary lesions can appear up to 5 months after vaccination.

In this clinical case, the patient had been treated with nonsteroidal anti-inflammatory drugs and subcutaneous enrofloxacin. Hair may regrow spontaneously, but this can take up to a year.

These lesions occur more frequently in the subcutaneous tissue of the neck and in small breeds. It is therefore recommended to avoid injection in this location in these breeds.

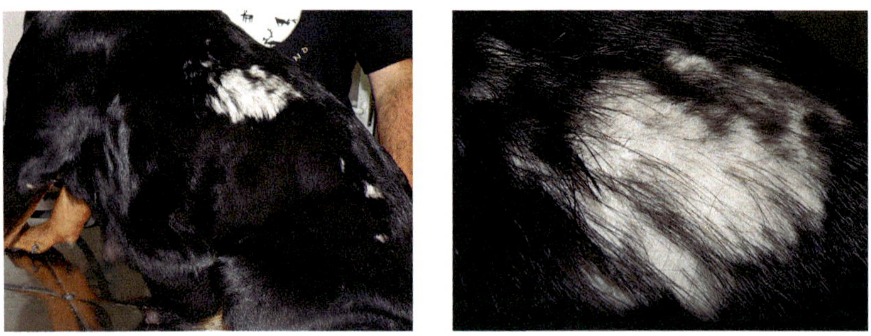

Figures 32.3 and 32.4. Bitch with multifocal alopecia with hypopigmentation caused by herpesvirus vaccine.

Case 33

Case presentation

A 5-year old male Bull Terrier was brought to our clinic with a cutaneous condition that had appeared 10 days earlier. The owner reported that the animal had been fitted with a deltamethrin-based insecticide collar, and 4 days later developed pruritic and painful exudative lesions on the dorsal aspect of the neck that rapidly and progressively extended to the trunk, head, and legs. His usual veterinary surgeon recommended antibiotic treatment with doxycycline at 10 mg/kg/day, baths with antiseptic shampoo, and removal of the insecticide collar. Despite the treatment, the lesions had not improved and the patient was dejected and anorexic. The pruritus was moderate. The patient had a clinical history of otitis externa, seasonal pododermatitis, and recurrent interdigital furunculosis with a good response to symptomatic treatment (cephalexin and topical therapy), but had no lesions of this type at the moment of consultation. Enlargement of the peripheral lymph nodes, fever, and prostration were observed in the general examination. In the dermatological examination, multiple diffuse alopecia, generalised crusted papular lesions, and pustular lesions on the inner aspect of the pinna were observed (Figs. 33.1–33.3). Cytology of the pustular lesions was carried out (Figs. 33.4 and 33.5).

Questions

1. What does the lesion cytology show?
2. What is the most probable diagnosis of this case, and how could it be confirmed?

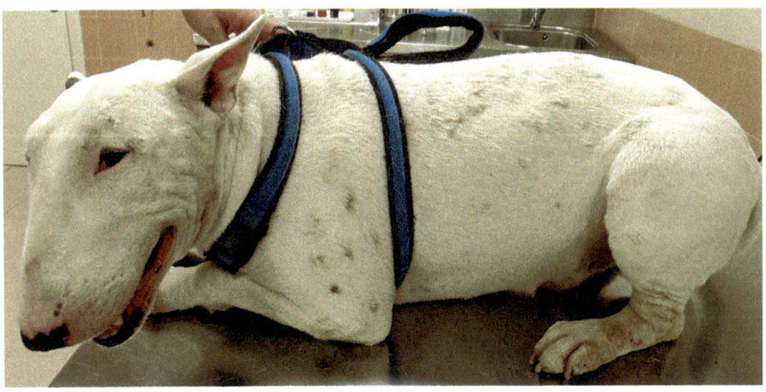

Figure 33.1. Multifocal alopecia with generalised crusted papular lesions.

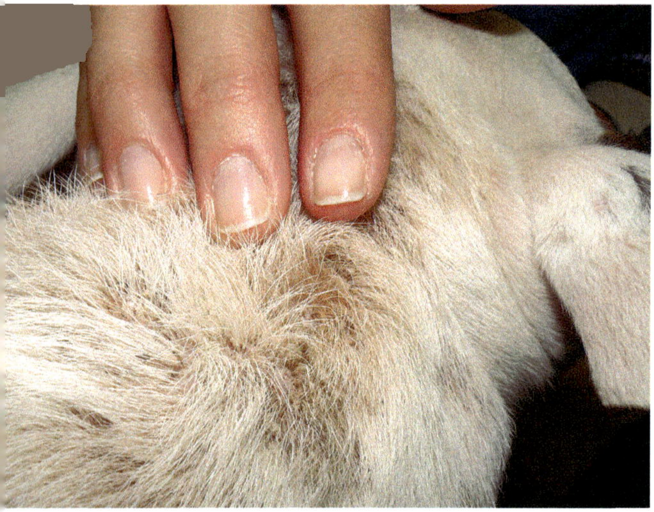

Figure 33.2. Detail of crusted papular skin lesions on the neck.

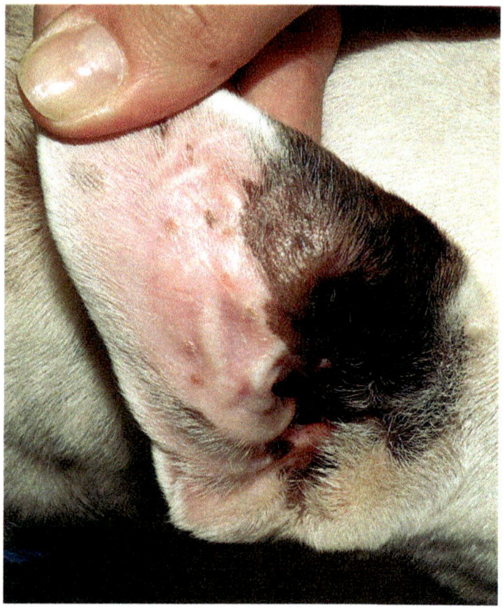

Figure 33.3. Pustular and crusted lesions on the inner aspect of the pinna.

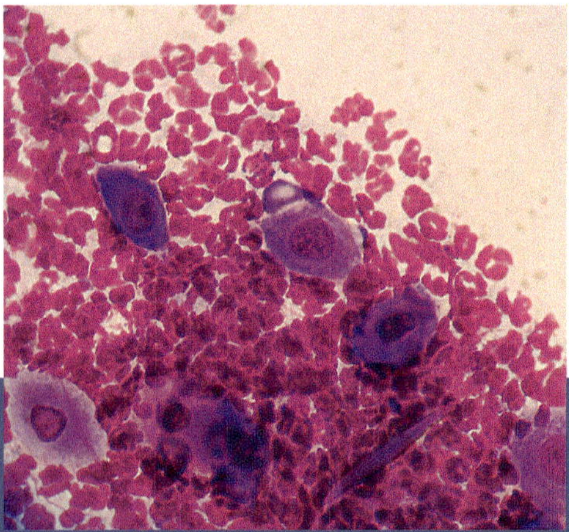

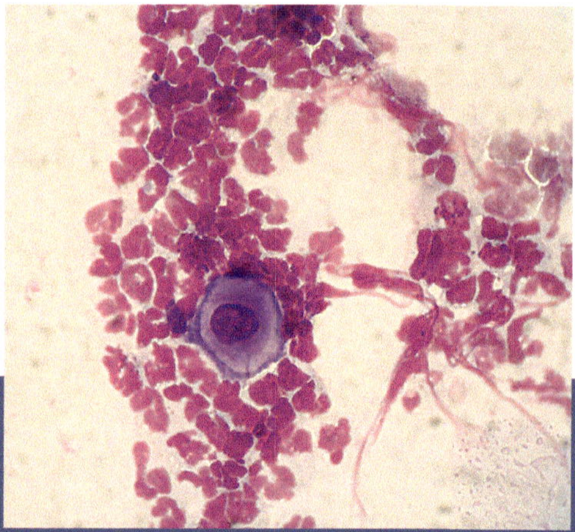

Figures 33.4 and 33.5. Cytology of the pustules showing polymorphonuclear neutrophils and acantholytic cells.

Answers Case 33

1 What does the lesion cytology show?

Cytology of the pustular lesions reveals the presence of numerous polymorphonuclear neutrophils and acantholytic keratinocytes. No infectious agents are evident.

2 What is the most probable diagnosis of this case, and how could it be confirmed?

The differential diagnosis in this case includes:

- Superficial pyoderma.
- Pemphigus foliaceus and other autoimmune diseases.
- Leishmaniasis.

Bacterial culture and serological tests for leishmaniasis were negative. Skin biopsy revealed histological changes similar to those observed in pemphigus foliaceus, with subcorneal pustules with neutrophils and acantholytic keratinocytes (Figs. 33.6 and 33.7).

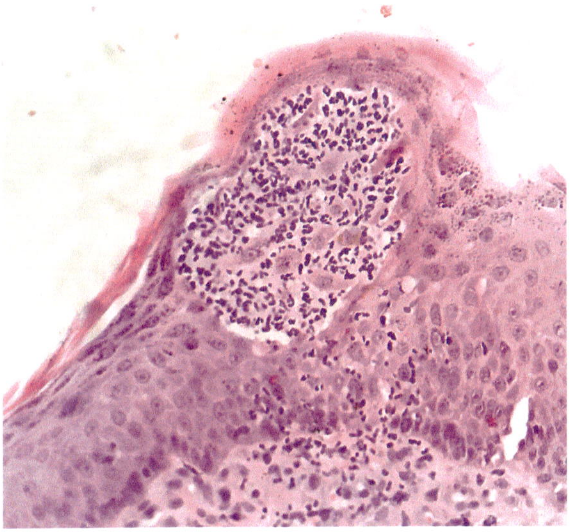

Figure 33.6. Subcorneal pustule with neutrophils and acantholytic cells typical of pemphigus foliaceus.

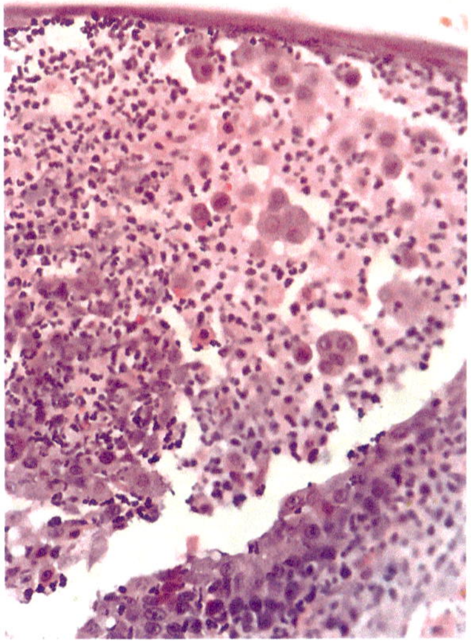

Figure 33.7. Detail of the pustular content in which acantholytic keratinocytes surrounded by neutrophils can be seen.

Observations

Canine pemphigus foliaceus (PF) is an autoimmune disease of the skin, usually of unknown aetiology. PF caused by the administration of certain medications is well described in human medicine but is very rare in veterinary medicine. In dogs, it can be associated with the administration of systemic medications, especially the combination of sulfadimethoxine and trimethoprim. Acantholytic pustular dermatitis similar to pemphigus foliaceus induced by the administration of metaflumizone and amitraz via pipette has also been described in dogs.

Deltamethrin (DTM) is an active substance belonging to the pyrethroid family. It exerts an intense and rapid insecticidal and acaricidal effect via direct contact or ingestion. After passing through the tegument of the parasite, it acts on the central nervous system. It is sold in a variety of different formulations for use in veterinary medicine. In the collar formulation, DTM is tightly bound to a triphenyl phosphate (TPP) excipient, forming a complex that is released progressively. Its main indications are the prevention of fleas, ticks, and phlebotomine bites in dogs. In this clinical case, deltamethrin and the triphenyl phosphate excipient may have triggered a PF-type drug reaction, similar to that described for metaflumizone + amitraz.

Case 34

Case presentation

A 2-month-old male kitten, who had been found in the street, was brought by his owners to the clinic with very poor condition hair and skin. The cat licked himself frequently. The general examination revealed no abnormalities, although the hair was matted with abundant white scales (Figs. 34.1 and 34.2). Crusted lesions were observed on the ear margins, the forehead, and the bridge of the nose. Brushing and skin scraping revealed the presence of a variety of parasites (Figs. 34.3 and 34.4).

Questions

1. What are these parasites?
2. What treatment would be appropriate?

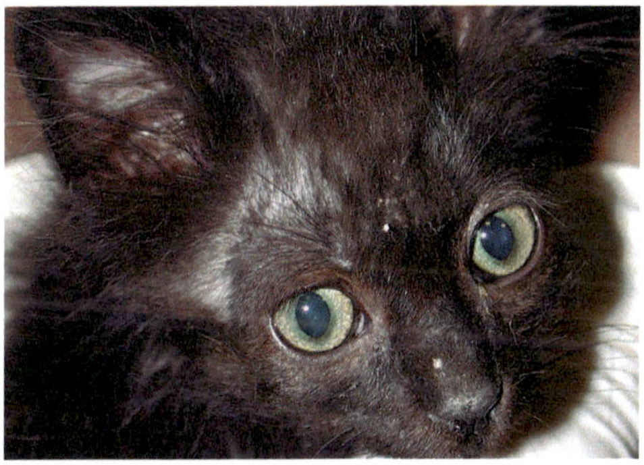

Figure 34.1. Keratoseborrhoeic lesions on the forehead, nasal bridge, and ear margin. Greyish-white scales are also evident.

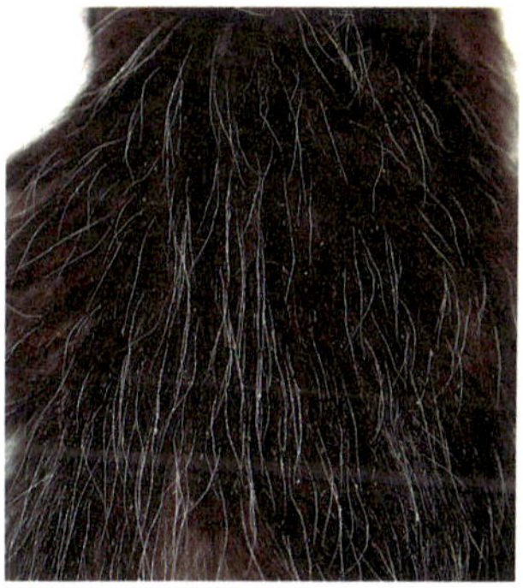

Figure 34.2. Scaling on the back and poor haircoat condition.

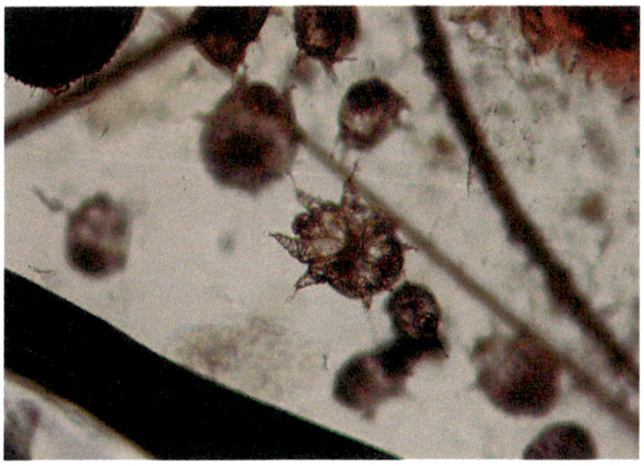

Figure 34.3. Skin scraping.

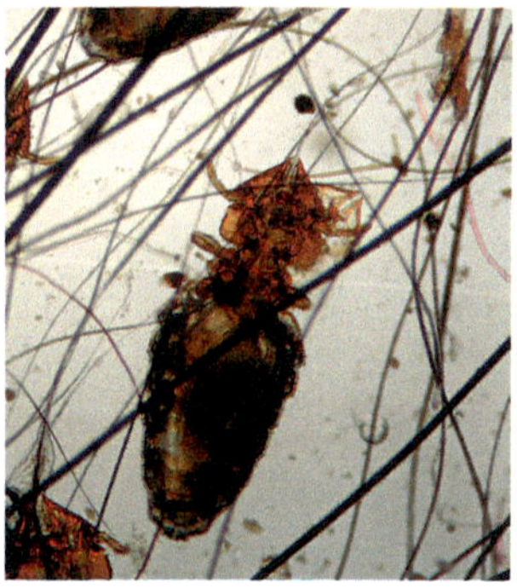

Figure 34.4. Material obtained by brushing.

Answers Case 34

1 What are these parasites?

The parasite in Figure 34.3 is a mite called *Notoedres cati*. Figure 34.4 shows a specific biting louse of cats called *Felicola subrostratus*.

Notoedric mange mainly affects wild cats and those housed in shelters. It causes highly pruritic keratoseborrhoeic lesions that affect the medial ear margin, face, neck, perineum, and limbs (Fig. 34.5).

Pediculosis is an infestation caused by a species-specific louse. It is uncommon and has been observed in neglected and malnourished young animals. Clinical signs include seborrhoea, alopecia, and secondary excoriations. The haircoat may be dense and matted. Nits (eggs) can be observed as whitish specks attached to the hair (Fig. 34.6).

2 What treatment would be appropriate?

In this case, the cat should be treated for the two parasitic conditions in question. The patient should be treated with subcutaneous ivermectin at 200–400 µg/kg, every 2 weeks, or selamectin by pipette every 2 weeks for 2 months.

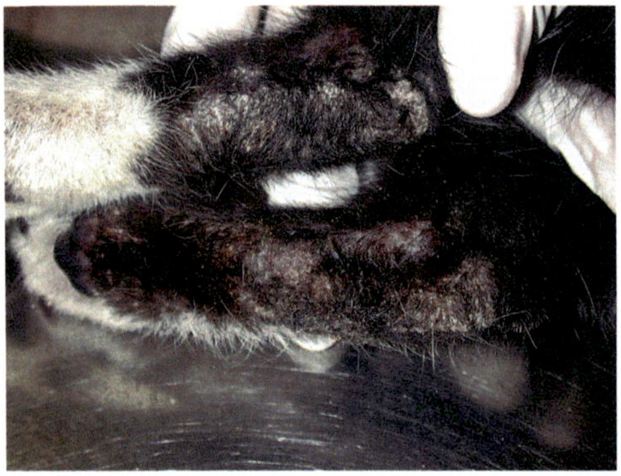

Figure 34.5. Seborrhoeic and crusted lesions on the limbs caused by notoedric mange.

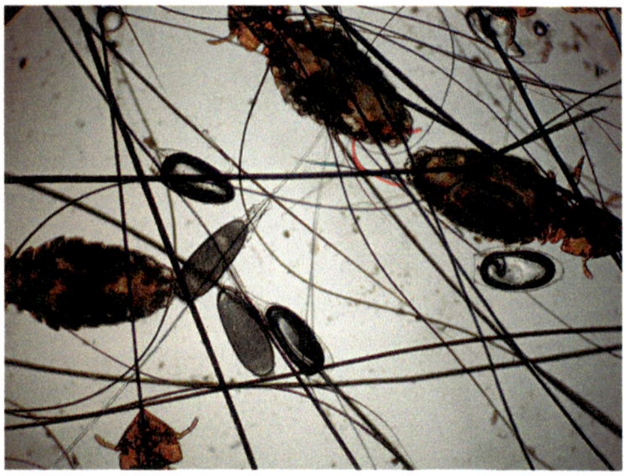

Figure 34.6. *Felicola subrostratus* and eggs (nits) attached to the hair.

Case 35

Case presentation

The patient, a 3-year-old, intact Collie bitch, had been licking the digits of her forepaws for a month. The owners reported no other clinical signs. The results of the general examination were normal. A change in hair colour from white to reddish brown was observed in the dermatological examination (Fig. 35.1). Erythema, exudation, and crusting were observed beneath the hair on the skin of the digits, as well as a dark exudate in the nail bed and discolouration of the nail itself (Fig. 35.2).

Questions

1. What could explain the appearance of a dark exudate around the nail?
2. Could this explain the intense pruritus?
3. How could the diagnosis be confirmed?

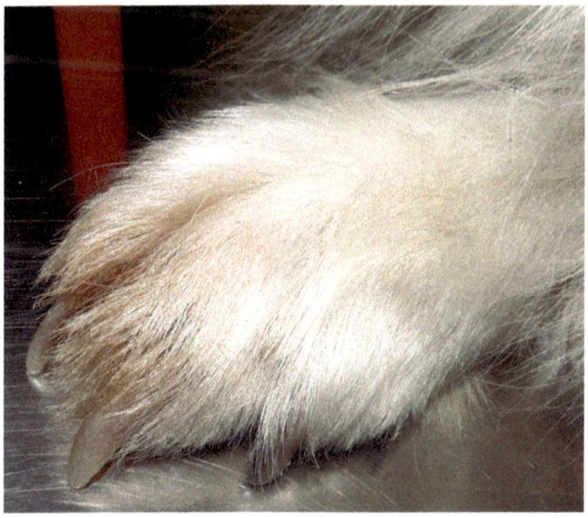

Figure 35.1. Change of hair colour on the digits.

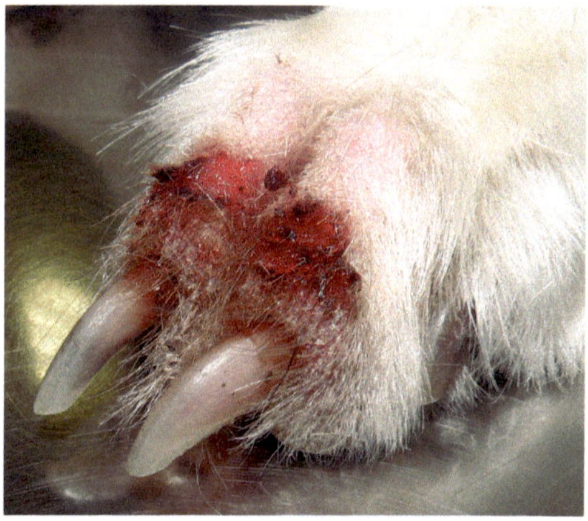

Figure 35.2. Image taken after clipping the hair of the digits. Note the erythema, crusting, and erosion of the skin, and the dark exudate around the nail, as well as the discolouration of the nail.

Answers Case 35

1 What could explain the appearance of a dark exudate around the nail?

The exudate may indicate an inflammatory process in the nail bed called paronychia. Inflammatory processes around the nail are usually associated with overgrowth of *Malassezia* spp. or bacteria. The change in colour from white hair to reddish could be due to saliva; porphyrins in the saliva have a staining effect on hair.

2 Could this explain the intense pruritus?

Paronychia due to *Malassezia* is very common in allergic dogs and is intensely pruritic. It is characterised by a dark exudate and brownish discolouration of the nail.

3 How could the diagnosis be confirmed?

A presumptive diagnosis can be confirmed by cytology of the exudate. In this case, overgrowth of *Malassezia* in the nail bed was evident, as well as a purulent exudate with crusted lesions on the digit secondary to constant licking and biting (Fig. 35.3).

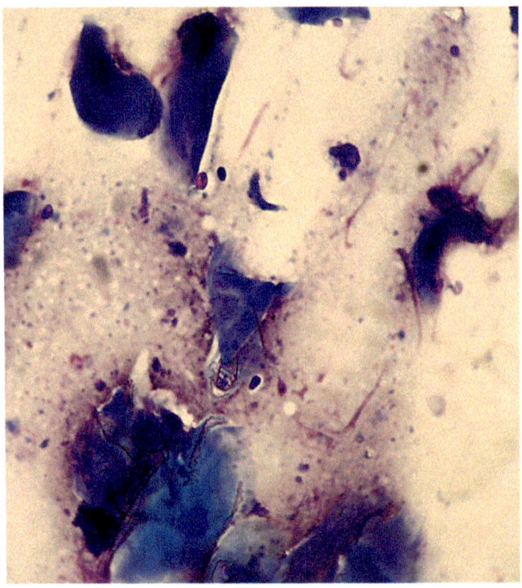

Figure 35.3. Exudate in which superficial epithelial cells and *Malassezia* spp. can be seen.

Case 36

Case presentation

The owners of a 20-month-old male Boxer came to our clinic to report the appearance of painful lumps in their dog's chin area that secreted a haemorrhagic fluid. The family had spent a few days on holiday in a house with a garden, and the dog had spent many hours outdoors.

The patient presented with papules, pustules, and nodules on the chin and upper lip (Fig. 36.1). The lesions were very painful and secreted a haemorrhagic exudate. The physical and dermatological examinations produced no other findings of note.

Questions

1 What pathologies should be included in the differential diagnosis of this clinical picture?

2 What tests would help establish the diagnosis?

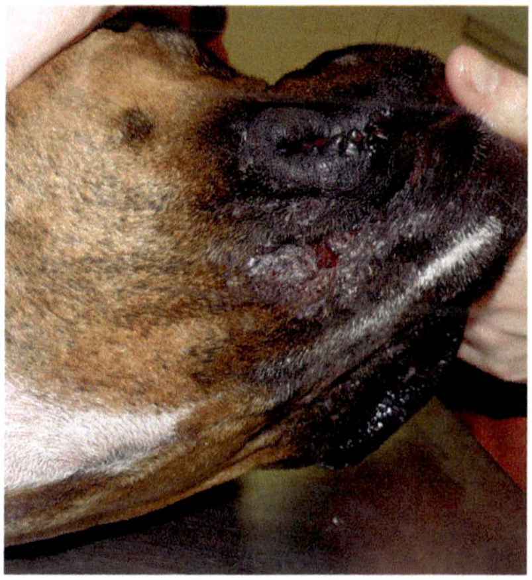

Figure 36.1. Nodules with haemorrhagic exudate in the chin area.

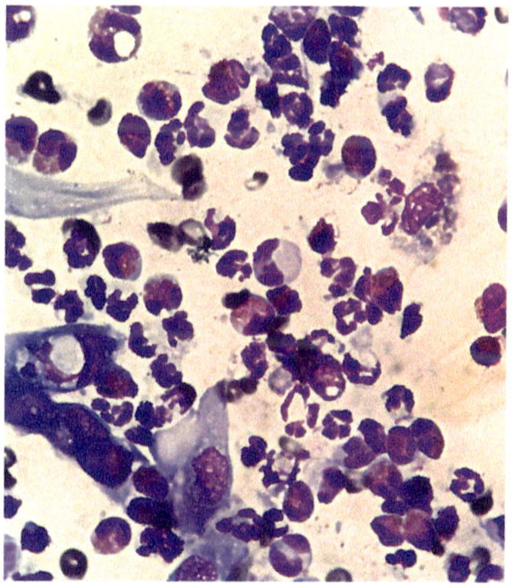

Figure 36.2. Cytological image of the haemorrhagic exudate.

Answers Case 36

1 What pathologies should be included in the differential diagnosis of this clinical picture?

The list of most likely diagnoses includes demodicosis, bacterial folliculitis-furunculosis, and eosinophilic folliculitis-furunculosis.

2 What tests would help establish the diagnosis?

The diagnostic protocol includes basic tests such as a trichogram and skin scraping, exudate cytology, and bacterial culture.

The results of the skin scraping and bacterial culture were negative. Cytology of the haemorrhagic exudate revealed numerous eosinophils and neutrophils and occasional macrophages (Fig. 36.2). The most probable diagnosis in this case is eosinophilic folliculitis-furunculosis.

Observations

Canine eosinophilic folliculitis-furunculosis is a rare disorder. Incidence is higher in young, active males, generally of large breeds (to date it has not been described in small or miniature breeds), who spend a lot of time outdoors. It has been proposed that this disorder is caused by a hypersensitivity reaction to the bites of arthropods, especially wasps and bees, although cases occurring during the winter months have been reported and attributed to spider bites. The lesions appear abruptly (within hours), and if not treated can persist for more than 3 weeks. The primary lesions are haemorrhagic vesicles or papules that progress to nodules and plaques that can ulcerate, bleed, or release exudate. Pruritus can range from intense to absent, but the lesions are usually very painful. They typically appear on the bridge of the nose or on the muzzle (Fig. 36.3), but less frequently can affect other locations such as the trunk, limbs, tips of the ears, lips, and eyelids. Cytology shows abundant eosinophils, and in some cases (due to a secondary bacterial infection) neutrophils with toxic changes containing bacteria within. Eosinophilia is usually observed in affected dogs.

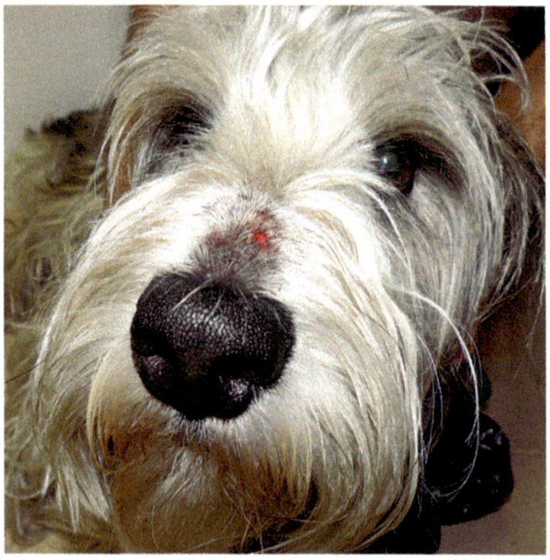

Figure 36.3. Eosinophilic furunculosis on the nasal bridge of a dog.

Treatment with systemic glucocorticoids is very effective, with most dogs showing a good response within 24 to 48 hours, and complete resolution of clinical signs within approximately 2 weeks of starting treatment.

Case 37

Case presentation

A 7-year-old male mongrel was brought to the clinic with a wound acquired 2 years earlier that had failed to properly heal. The wound caused him to limp. Despite the administration of different topical treatments by the owner, nothing appeared to work. The dog was eating well and his general condition was good. He never licked the wound.

The patient was underweight (body condition, 5/10). The examination revealed no other findings of note.

Inflammation of the second digit of the left forepaw was observed in the dermatological examination. There was a large ulcer in the centre of the footpad (Fig. 37.1). The wound exuded and contained a short fistulous tract. The dog showed signs of pain on palpation of the digit.

Radiography of the digits of the affected limb showed soft-tissue inflammation with no bone or joint lesions (Fig. 37.2). Cytology of the exudate of the ulcer revealed a pyogranulomatous inflammatory pattern.

Questions

1. What pathologies should be included in the differential diagnosis of the lesions on this dog's digit?
2. What other diagnostic tests would be indicated?

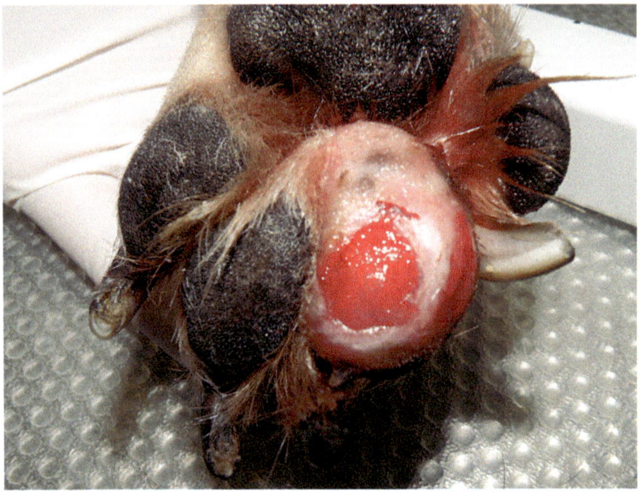

Figure 37.1. Inflamed and swollen digit with large central ulcer.

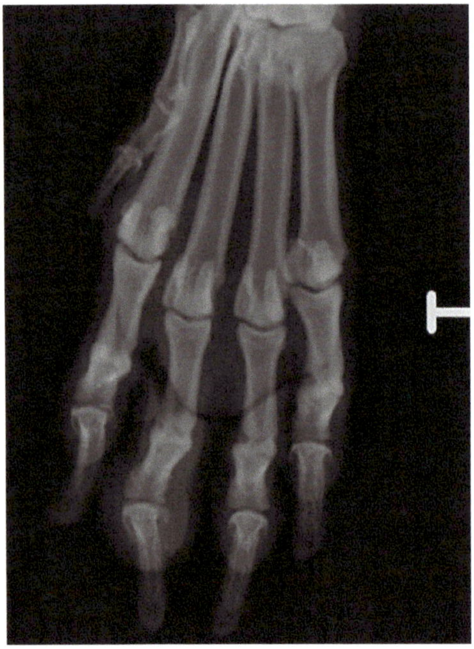

Figure 37.2. Radiograph of the limb showing soft-tissue inflammation.

Answers Case 37

1 What pathologies should be included in the differential diagnosis of the lesions on this dog's digit?

This dog presented with the following problems: poor body condition; inflammation and pain in a digit with an indolent ulcer; lameness with no apparent bone lesions; and pyogranulomatous inflammatory exudate in the affected area.

The differential diagnosis consisted of the following:

- Granuloma due to a foreign body.
- Deep pyoderma.
- Granuloma due to atypical bacteria.
- *Leishmania* granuloma.

The possibility that the lesion was a soft tissue neoplasm (squamous cell carcinoma, fibrosarcoma) was less likely.

Taking into account the differential diagnosis, culture and antibiogram of the exudate were performed. *Staphylococcus pseudintermedius* sensitive to quinolone antibiotics grew in the culture. Treatment with oral ciprofloxacin at 10 mg/kg every 12 hours was initiated and the wound was protected with a bandage.

Ten days later, the dog showed less pain, but the digit was still very inflamed and the lesion remained ulcerated.

2 What other diagnostic tests would be indicated?

Given the poor response to symptomatic treatment, it was recommended that the dog undergo a biopsy under general anaesthesia.

In the preoperative analyses, blood tests showed moderate anaemia, severe thrombocytopaenia, and hypergammaglobulinaemia. Suspecting an infectious cause, serological tests for leishmaniasis and ehrlichiosis were performed, as well as bone marrow cytology. Amastigotes of *Leishmania infantum* were detected in the bone marrow and antibody titres (1/400, indirect immunofluorescence) were positive for leishmaniasis (Fig. 37.3).

The patient was treated with antimonial compounds and allopurinol. Thirty days after starting treatment, the ulcer had healed and the inflammation and pain in the digit had disappeared (Fig. 37.4). The dog began to recover weight.

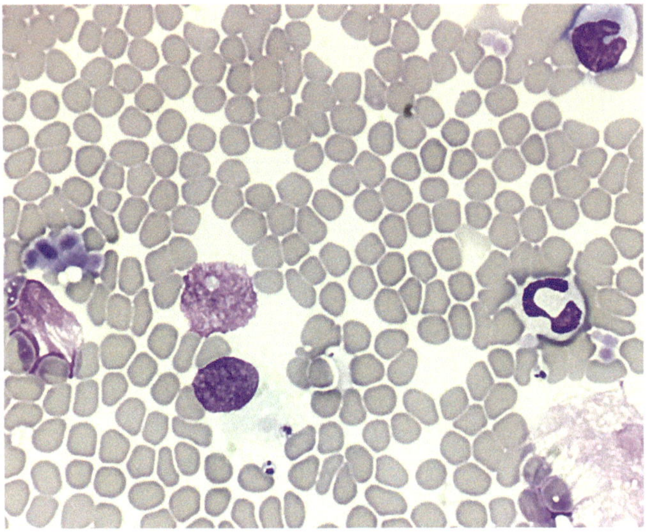

Figure 37.3. Macrophage containing amastigotes of *Leishmania* spp.

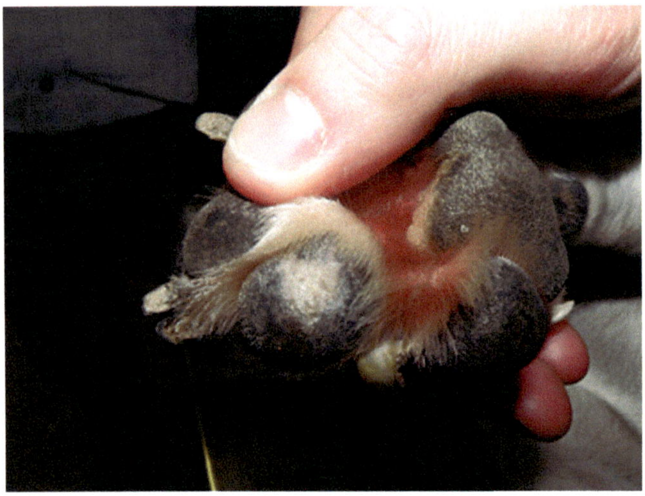

Figure 37.4. Appearance of the digit 30 days after beginning treatment for leishmaniasis.

Case 38

Case presentation

Different types of fungi are shown in Figures 38.1–38.4.

Questions

1 Based on their morphology, which are pathogens and which are the result of contamination?

2 How should these samples be prepared for microscopic observation?

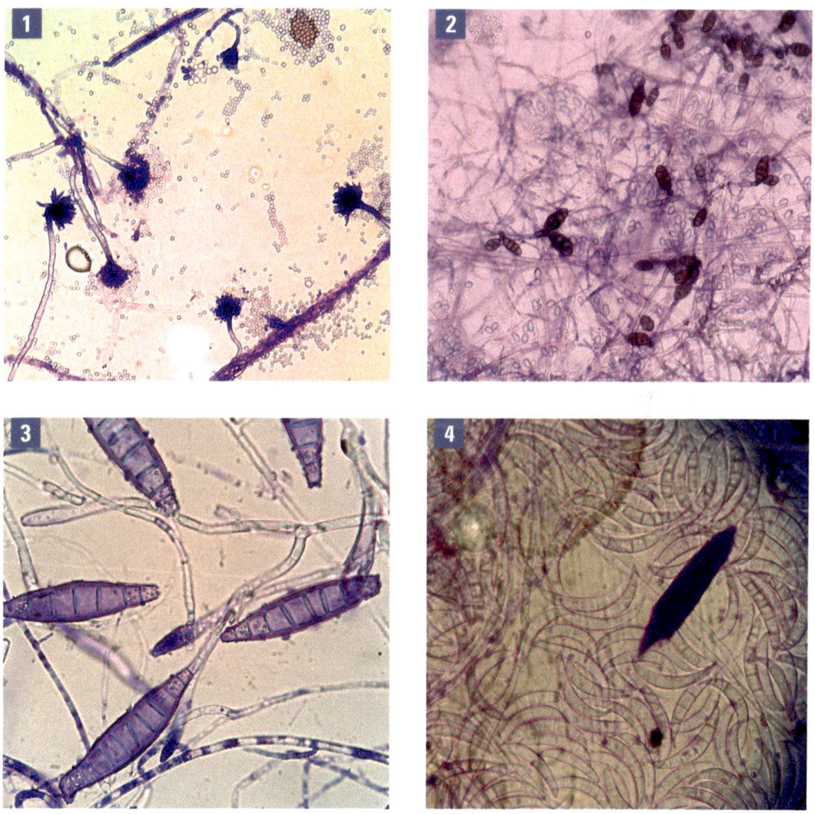

Figures 38.1–38.4. Conidia of different fungi.

Answers Case 38

1 Which are pathogens and which are the result of contamination?

Figure 38.1 shows conidia of *Aspergillus* spp. Figure 38.2 shows conidia of *Alternaria* spp. Figure 38.3 shows macroconidia of *Microsporum canis and* Figure 38.4 macroconidia of *Fusarium* spp.

Alternaria is a saprophytic and contaminating fungus. *Aspergillus* and *Fusarium* are usually saprophytic fungi, although they can sometimes cause skin lesions. *M. canis* is a pathogenic dermatophyte with zoonotic potential. In general, contaminating fungi are more pigmented than dermatophytes.

The macroconidia of *M. canis* are canoe-shaped, with six or more cells and a thick wall (Fig. 38.5). The conidia of *M. gypseum* contain less than six cells and have a thin wall.

2 How should these samples be prepared for microscopic observation?

To identify the fungi under the microscope a strip of adhesive tape is pressed onto the growing colony. A drop of blue dye is placed on the slide and the strip of tape is placed on top and viewed under a microscope.

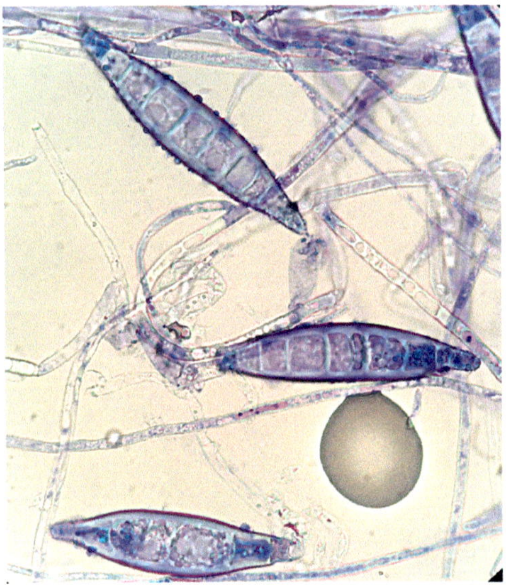

Figure 38.5. Macroconidia of *Microsporum canis.*

Case 39

Case presentation

The owners of a 7-year-old mongrel dog brought him to the emergency veterinary service with acute pruritus affecting the anal area. The dog licked himself continuously and dragged his hindquarters along the ground. Examination revealed erythema around the anus and at the base of the tail, as well as a brown and haemorrhagic exudate at the 5 o'clock position relative to the anus (Fig. 39.1).

Questions

1. Based on the clinical signs and the results of the examination, what pathology is suggested?
2. What treatment would be appropriate?

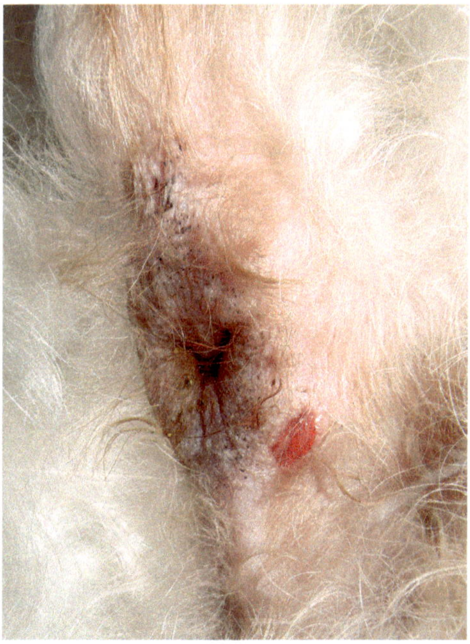

Figure 39.1. Appearance of the anal area of the patient.

Answers Case 39

1 Based on the clinical signs and the results of the examination, what pathology is suggested?

The clinical picture is highly suggestive of anal sacculitis. Most carnivores have anal sacs. These are modified skin appendages that form a stratified squamous epithelium. They serve as a reservoir for a set of apocrine and sebaceous glands, the contents of which drain into the keratinised portion of this epithelium. The variation in the secretions of these apocrine and sebaceous glands, in addition to other constituents of the anal sac, such as the metabolic products of bacteria and yeasts, can alter the consistency of the exudate, hindering emptying of the contents and resulting in anal gland impaction. Anal sac disorders are classified as follows: impaction, inflammation, and infection.

The clinical signs are related to the painful condition produced by distension of the anal sac and the irritation caused by inflammation and secondary infection. Typical signs include anal licking, nibbling under the tail, and dragging of the hindquarters. These may be accompanied by tenesmus, painful defecation, self-injury of the tail, and perineal pyotraumatic dermatitis. In cases involving abscesses perianal erythema, inflammation, fistulous tracts (if the abscess ruptures), and fever may be observed (Fig. 39.2).

2 What treatment would be appropriate?

Treatment of impaction consists of manual emptying of the anal sacs. The best way to do this is to express them by anorectal examination. In the case of sacculitis, in addition to emptying, the anal sacs should be washed with 0.025 % chlorhexidine solution and then treated with an antibiotic/glucocorticoid cream (Figs. 39.3 and 39.4). Abscesses of the anal sacs should be drained and the anal sacs washed as described above. Treatment with systemic broad-spectrum antibiotics for 7 or 14 days is recommended in cases of both sacculitis and abscesses.

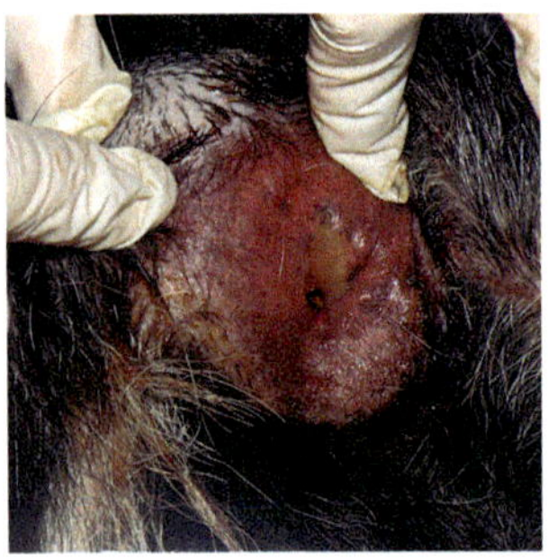

Figure 39.2. Ruptured abscess of the anal sac with a fistulous tract.

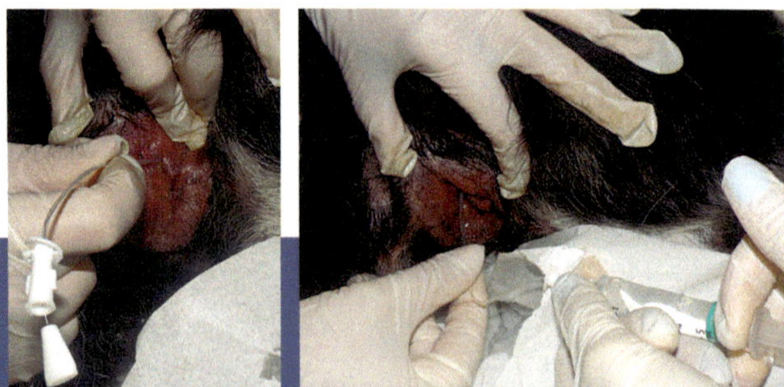

Figures 39.3 and 39.4. Washing of the anal sacs.

Case 40

Case presentation

A pair of 10-month-old goats that had been donated to a veterinary teaching hospital developed an acute episode of intense pruritus. The two goats presented with similar lesions, consisting of mild erythema, marked dry scaling, and exfoliation affecting the muzzle, pinnae, and to a lesser extent the rest of the body (Figs. 40.1 and 40.2).

Questions

1. What type of dermatological pattern is observed in these animals?
2. Could this be a contagious process?

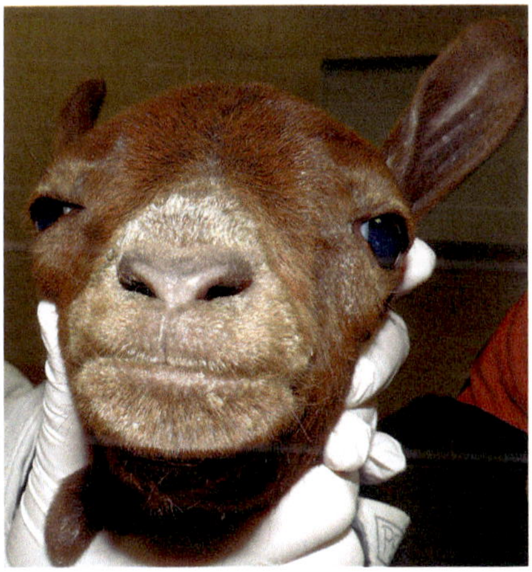

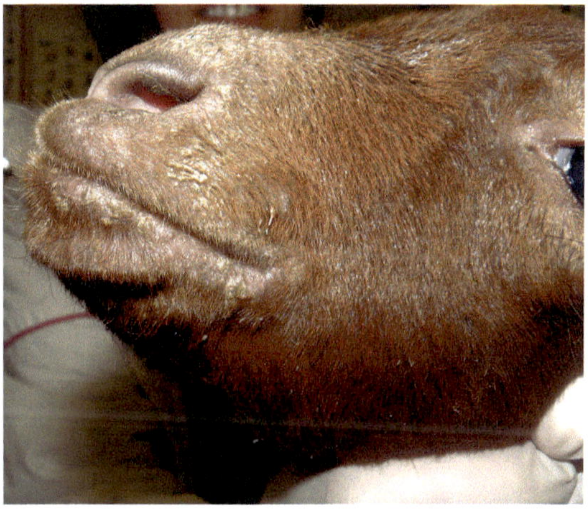

Figures 40.1 and 40.2. Flaking and exfoliation on the muzzle and pinna of one of the goats.

Answers Case 40

1 What type of dermatological pattern is observed in these animals?

The dermatological pattern is that of an exfoliative keratoseborrhoeic process.

2 Could this be a contagious process?

Given that this case of pruritus was, in theory, contagious (since the two animals presented with the same clinical signs), parasitosis and dermatophytosis were included in the initial differential diagnosis. Multiple skin scrapings and trichograms were negative for parasites, and no fungal arthrospores were detected. Lesion cytology showed an exudate composed mainly of large numbers of neutrophils, with occasional macrophages and some acantholytic cells (Fig. 40.3). Moderate amounts of *Malassezia* were also evident. Seborrhoeic and exfoliative dermatitis in goats has been attributed to *Malassezia* spp.

In this case, culture in DTM medium was performed, and while awaiting the results the goats were bathed with a shampoo containing 2 % chlorhexidine. The response to treatment was very good, with almost complete resolution of the lesions and pruritus after the first bath (Figs. 40.4 and 40.5). The DTM culture was negative.

Malassezia infection should be included in the differential diagnosis of seborrhoeic and exfoliative dermatitis in goats. The *Malassezia* species that affect goats are difficult to grow. Therefore, cytological examination of the skin is a more effective means of identifying the organism.

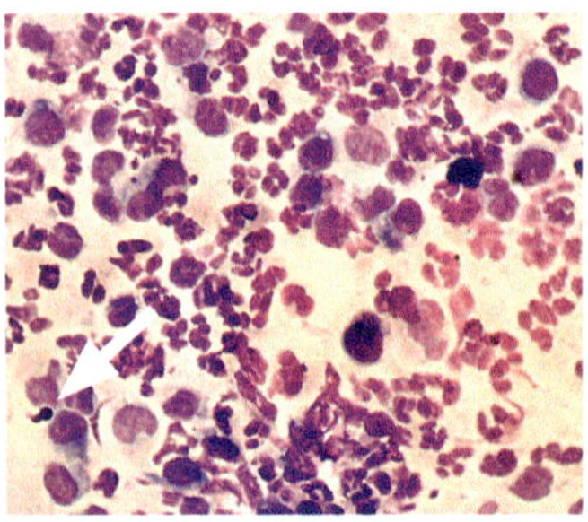

Figure 40.3. Exudate containing abundant neutrophilic granulocytes with toxic changes and macrophages in moderate numbers. Note the presence of *Malassezia* spp. (arrow).

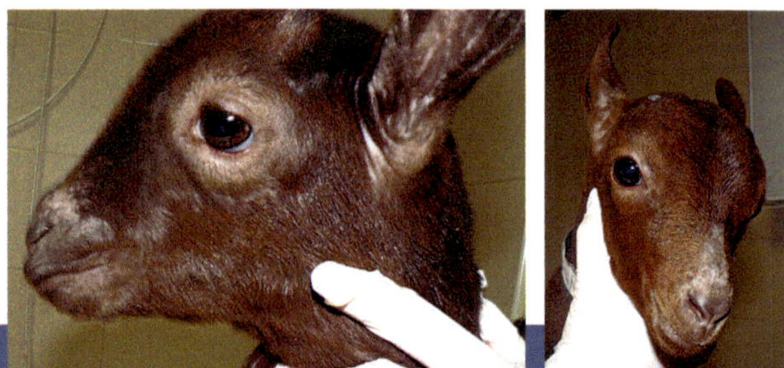

Figures 40.4 and 40.5. Appearance of goats 8 days after starting treatment with a 2 % chlorhexidine shampoo. Almost complete resolution of the lesions is observed.

Case 41

Case presentation

The owners of an intact male Shar Pei of 1.5 years of age brought him to the dermatology clinic with a pruritic condition that was associated with hair loss and a bad odour, and had appeared about 4 months earlier. The dog had been treated with corticosteroids and antibiotics, but showed only a partial response. The patient exhibited aggression.

His general condition was good, except for mild lymphadenopathy and a bilateral blepharospasm caused by a congenital entropion.

The skin examination revealed erythema, exudation, hyperpigmentation, alopecia, and hyperkeratosis on the face, pinnae, ventral aspect of the neck, and axillae, and multifocal alopecia on the trunk (Figs. 41.1–41.3). Excoriations were observed in the axillary area (Fig. 41.3). Erythema, alopecia, and hyperpigmentation were also observed in the distal portion of the limbs. All lesions were highly exudative.

Questions

1 What differential diagnoses do these clinical signs suggest?

2 What diagnostic tests should be performed?

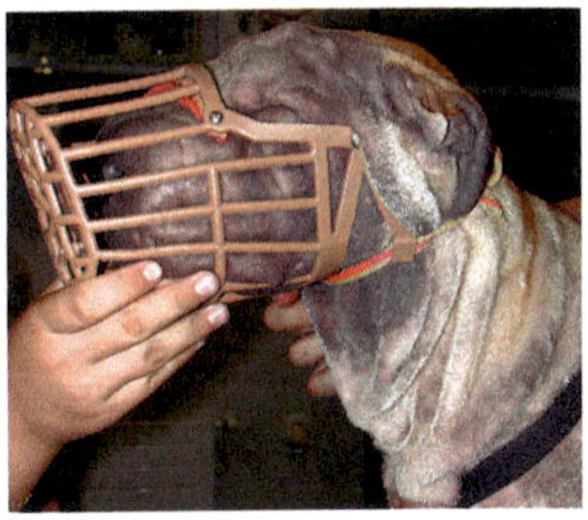

Figure 41.1. Alopecia, erythema, hyperpigmentation, and lichenification on the face, pinna, and ventral aspect of the neck.

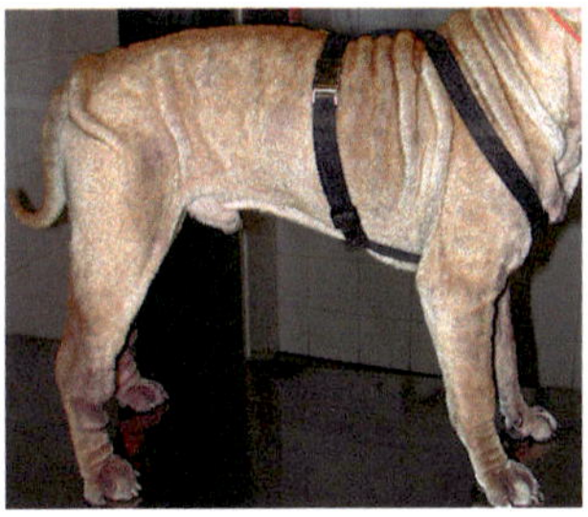

Figure 41.2. Multifocal alopecia on the trunk and alopecia with hyperpigmentation on the distal portions of the limbs.

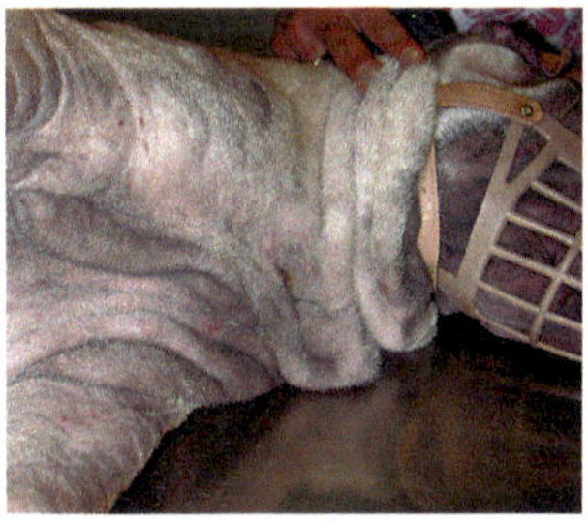

Figure 41.3. Hyperpigmentation and exudation on the ventral aspect of the body. Excoriations secondary to pruritus are evident.

Answers Case 41

1 What differential diagnoses do these clinical signs suggest?

Exudative and foul-smelling lesions suggest an inflammatory process with secondary infection. Inflammatory multifocal alopecia can be caused by superficial pyoderma, bacterial or *Malassezia* overgrowth, demodicosis, or dermatophytosis.

2 What diagnostic tests should be performed?

In this case, multiple skin scrapings proved negative. Samples for cytological analysis were taken by swabbing and by direct impression on the neck, abdomen, axillae, and limbs.

In all cases the same profile was observed: numerous bacteria (cocci), superficial epithelial cells, and some polymorphonuclear neutrophils (Fig. 41.4).

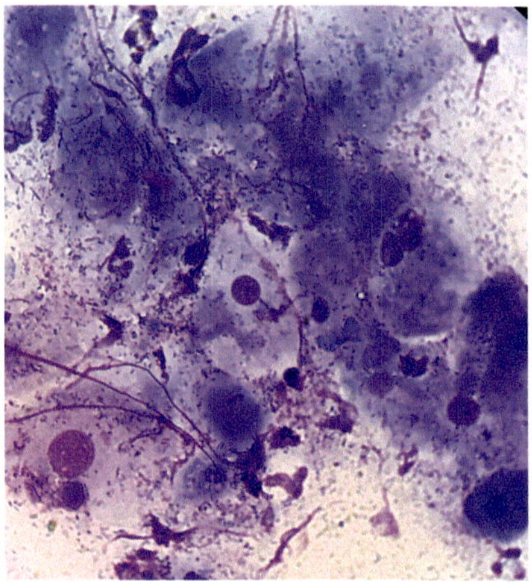

Figure 41.4. Skin surface cytology, in which superficial epithelial cells and numerous bacteria adhered to the keratinocytes are observed.

Observations

Microbial overgrowth is a syndrome caused by colonisation of the skin by microorganisms. The most common aetiologic agents are coagulase-positive staphylococci and the yeast *Malassezia*.

Bacterial overgrowth is a recently documented syndrome that is caused by the widespread proliferation of *Staphylococcus pseudintermedius* on the surface of the skin, without deep lesions. It usually affects young dogs, and is characterised by intense pruritus, erythema, lichenification, exudation, oily seborrhoea, and bad odour. Lesion distribution is variable, and can be localised (e.g. ventral aspect of the neck), regional (abdomen), or more or less generalised, although the ventral area of the body is predominantly affected. Clinically, the main characteristic of bacterial overgrowth is the absence of papules, pustules, and collarettes, since bacteria are found on the surface of the skin, not in the hair follicle.

In most cases bacterial overgrowth syndrome is associated with primary allergic processes. The differential diagnosis is broad, and includes parasitic diseases such as demodicosis, *Malassezia* dermatitis, and chronic allergic processes.

Case 42

Case presentation

A 2-year-old male German Shepherd was brought to the emergency room of the veterinary hospital with acute unilateral epistaxis and lesions on the nostrils and muzzle (Figs. 42.1 and 42.2).

Questions

1. What lesions are evident on the right nostril and the muzzle?
2. What is the most likely diagnosis of this clinical picture, and what could be the underlying cause?

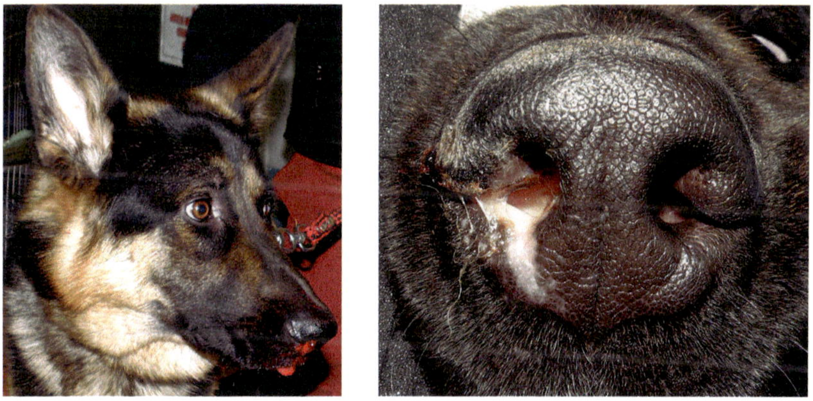

Figures 42.1 and 42.2. Patient with unilateral epistaxis and appearance of the lesions on the nostrils and muzzle.

Answers Case 42

1 What lesions are evident on the right nostril and the muzzle?

Figure 42.1 shows a haemorrhage in the right nasal orifice. Blood masks the lesions on the muzzle. Figure 42.2 shows mucosal nasal exudate, crusts, and unilateral depigmentation of the muzzle.

2 What is the most likely diagnosis of this clinical picture, and what could be the underlying cause?

Unilateral nasal depigmentation associated with epistaxis is characteristic of nasal aspergillosis. Nasal aspergillosis is caused by saprophytic fungi that are distributed throughout the environment. Inhalation of the spores, usually associated with entry of a foreign body, causes a local infection and invasion of the nasal cavity and frontal sinuses. The skin lesions consist of inflammation, depigmentation, ulceration and crust formation in the nostrils and, occasionally, the nasal plane. The differential diagnosis should include other infectious diseases (leishmaniasis), immune-mediated diseases, nasal pyoderma, neoplasms, and drug eruption.

On suspicion of nasal aspergillosis, rhinoscopy was performed, revealing the presence of a spike in the nasal sinus, as well as necrotic tissue (Figs. 42.3 and 42.4). Cytology showed purulent exudate with numerous bacteria (cocci) and fungal spores and hyphae (Fig. 42.5). Serology and a biopsy confirmed infection by *Aspergillus fumigatus*.

During the endoscopy, the foreign body was removed and the affected tissue was cleaned. The patient was treated with topical enilconazole and oral itraconazole for 6 weeks, and had fully recovered within 6 months of finishing treatment (Fig. 42.6).

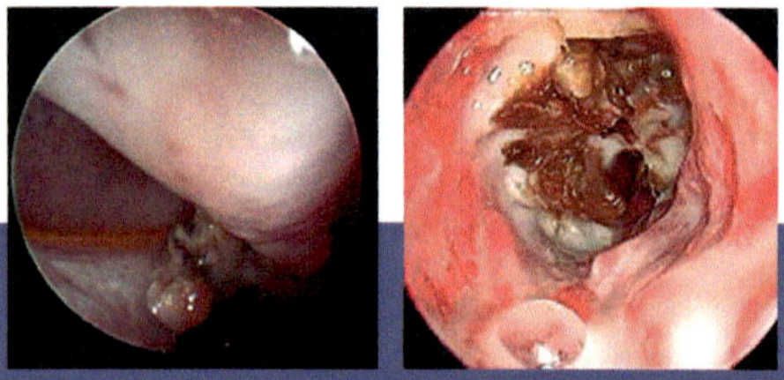

Figures 42.3 and 42.4. Images obtained by rhinoscopy showing necrotic tissue and a foreign body (spike).

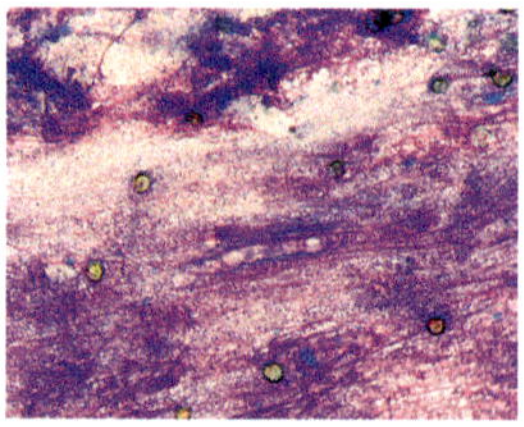

Figure 42.5. Exudate cytology showing fungal hyphae and bacterial overgrowth.

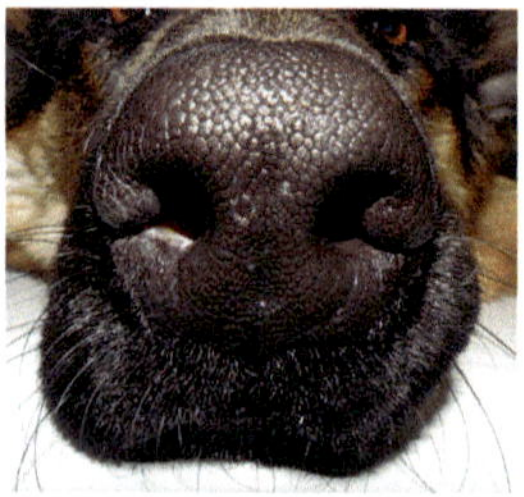

Figure 42.6. Appearance of the patient's muzzle 3 months after beginning treatment.

Case 43

Case presentation

A 12-year-old castrated male Poodle was brought to the clinic by his owner, who reported that she had detected black spots around her dog's anus (Fig. 43.1). The dog appeared unperturbed by the lesions. These lesions had appeared 4 months earlier, at which time the dog also had alopecia due to a testicular tumour (Fig. 43.2). The alopecia had resolved with castration of the animal, whereas the black spots had improved slightly, but had not disappeared.

Questions

1. What skin lesions are observed?
2. What could be the underlying cause?

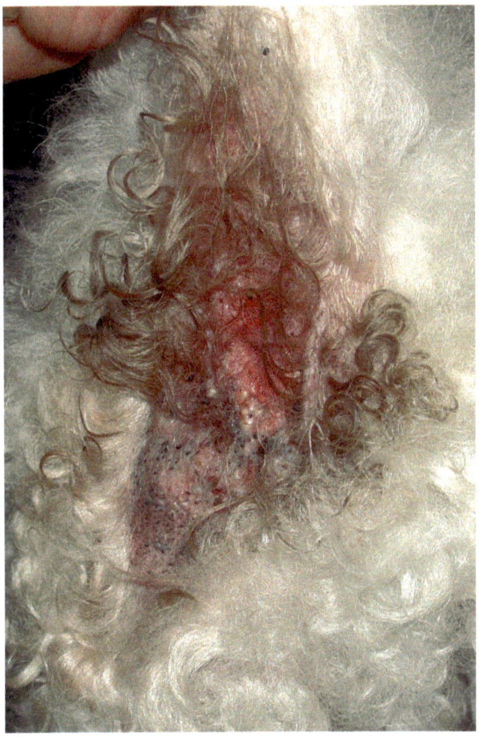

Figure 43.1. Lesions around the patient's anus.

Answers Case 43

1 What skin lesions are observed?

The lesions presented by this dog are comedones and milia.

2 What could be the underlying cause?

Comedones are caused by the accumulation of keratin in the follicular orifice. The white lesions (milia) are accumulations of keratin with no external opening, hence the paler colour. Comedones are primary lesions in endocrine diseases such as hyperadrenocorticism and sex hormone imbalance, in primary seborrhoea, Schnauzer comedone syndrome, and in vitamin A-responsive dermatosis, and appear secondarily in cases of demodicosis, dermatophytosis, and in response to occlusive topical treatment. Milia appear on the skin of dogs in response to an excess of glucocorticoids, either spontaneously or following parenteral or topical glucocorticoid administration. In this case, the skin scraping was negative for *Demodex*. Given the age and breed of the dog, a diagnostic protocol for hyperadrenocorticism was recommended.

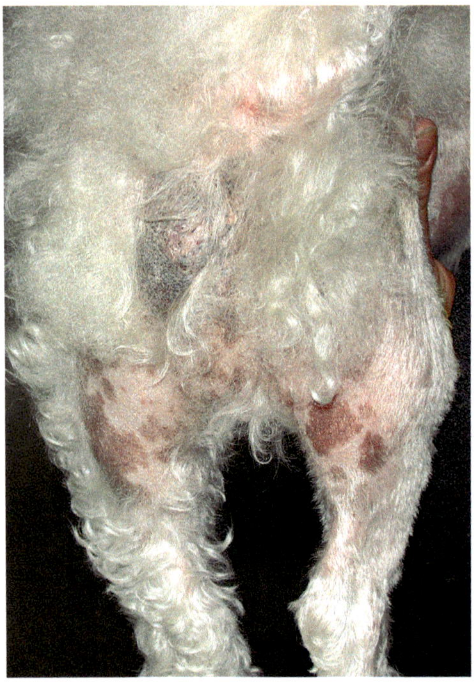

Figure 43.2. Perineal alopecia due to a testicular tumour with excessive production of oestrogen. Black spots around the anus are also evident.

Case 44

Case presentation

The following images correspond to hairs observed under the microscope (trichogram or trichography) (Figs. 44.1–44.4).

Questions

1 To which pathologies do these images correspond?

2 In what other pathologies is trichography useful?

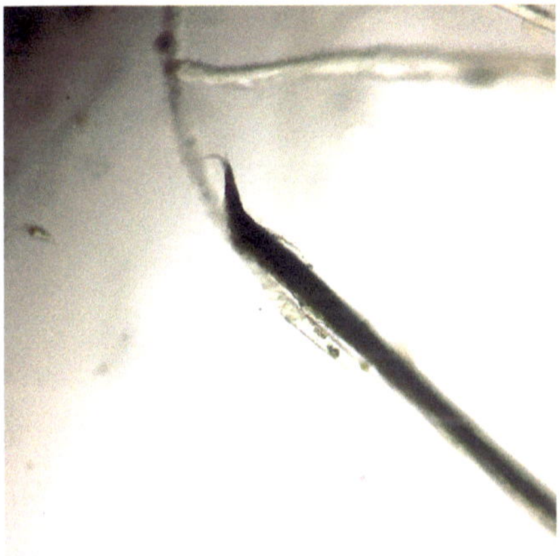

Figure 44.1.

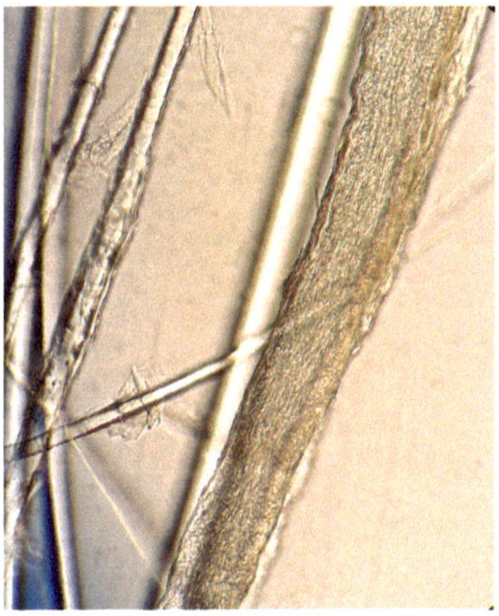

Figure 44.2.

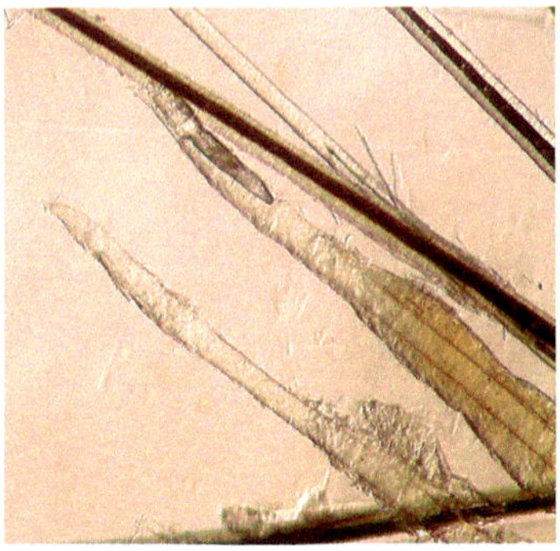

Figure 44.3.

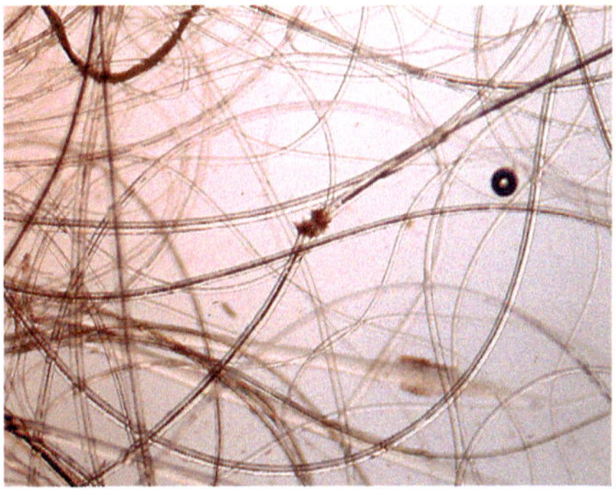

Figure 44.4.

Answers Case 44

1 To which pathologies do these images correspond?

In Figure 44.1, the hair tip shaped like an exclamation mark is characteristic of alopecia areata.

Figure 44.2 shows the hair of a dog with dermatophytosis. The diaphysis of the hair is distorted and oedematous, and numerous arthroconidia are evident.

In Figure 44.3 the body of an adult *Demodex* is observed on the hair root.

Figure 44.4 corresponds to trichorrhexis nodosa. The hair fractures, leaving the ends splayed, resembling two brooms pushed end to end.

2 In what other pathologies is trichography useful?

Microscopic observation of plucked hair is useful for the diagnosis of the following processes:

- Self-induced alopecia in cats.
- Dermatophytosis.
- Colour dilution alopecia.
- Congenital and acquired follicular dysplasias.
- Trichorrhexis nodosa.
- Trichoptilosis.
- Trichomalacia.
- Pili torti.
- Telogen effluvium.
- Demodicosis.

Case 45

Case presentation

A 1-year-old neutered male Persian cat was brought to the clinic with crusts on his face and pruritus. The owners also reported loss of hair on the back and on the thighs, and changes in hair colour in some areas. They had adopted the cat a month and a half earlier because his previous, elderly owner was no longer able to care for him. He lived with five other cats and appeared to be in good health. The owners did not have any skin lesions. Immediately after his adoption he had been tested for leukaemia and feline immunodeficiency virus, with negative results. The cat's general condition was good, and he had been properly vaccinated and dewormed. He lived exclusively indoors.

Crusted papular lesions with excoriations were observed in the preauricular area (Fig. 45.1). Otoscopy revealed the presence of ceruminous material and dark exudate in the ear canal (Fig. 45.2). The patient had hypotrichosis in the dorsal area of the trunk, with a change in colouration of the black hairs to reddish (Fig. 45.3), as well as alopecia in the perianal area, the posterior aspect of the thighs, and the base of the tail (Fig. 45.4).

Questions

1. List the problems presented by this cat.
2. What pathologies should be included in the differential diagnosis?
3. What diagnostic tests would you perform?

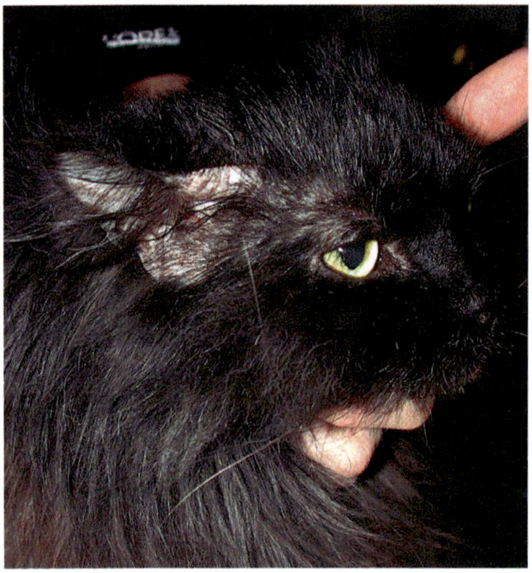

Figure 45.1. Crusts and excoriations in the preauricular area.

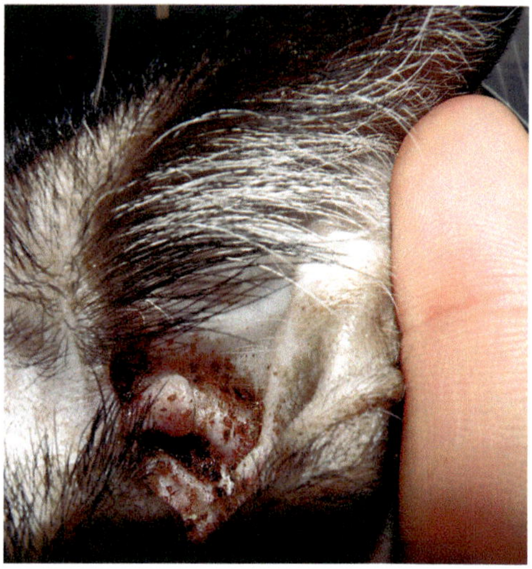

Figure 45.2. Dark exudate in the ear canal.

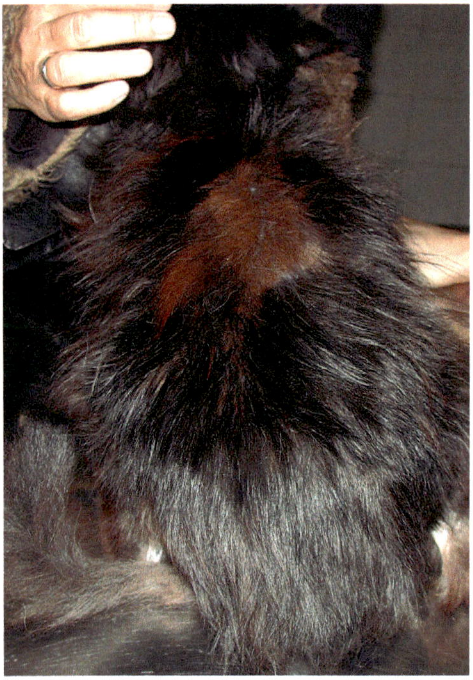

Figure 45.3. Hypotrichosis and changes in the colour of black hair to red.

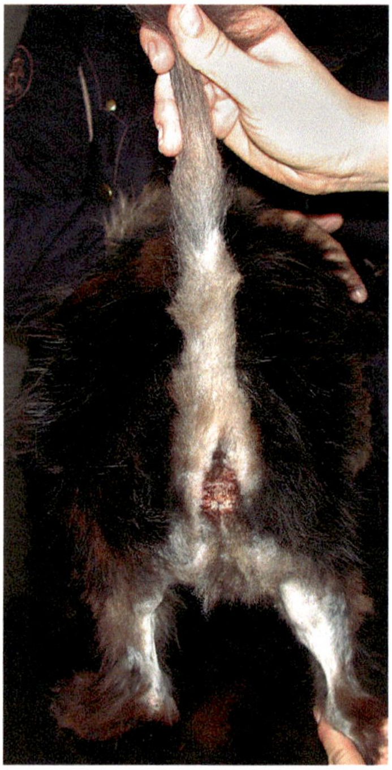

Figure 45.4. Alopecia around the anus, on the backs of the thighs, and at the base of the tail.

Answers Case 45

1 List the problems presented by this cat.

The patient presents the following lesions:

- Facial excoriations and crusts.
- Bilateral erythema and exudation in the ear canal.
- Hypotrichosis on the back.
- Alopecia in the perianal area and the posterior aspects of the thighs.
- Change in hair colour on the back.

2 What pathologies should be included in the differential diagnosis?

The clinical signs presented by this patient appear to be secondary to a pruritic condition, which could be caused by a hypersensitivity disorder, ectoparasites, dermatophytosis, or a bacterial or viral infection.

3 What diagnostic tests would you perform?

The initial diagnostic protocol should consist of brushing, skin scraping, a trichogram, and cytology of the otic exudate. The brushing and skin scraping revealed no parasites or flea droppings. No parasites or fungal spores were observed in the trichogram. Analysis of hair bulbs revealed a mixture of anagen and telogen hairs. The tips of some hairs were broken, with fractured diaphyses (Fig. 45.5). Mites of the genus *Otodectes* were observed in the otic exudate (Fig. 45.6).

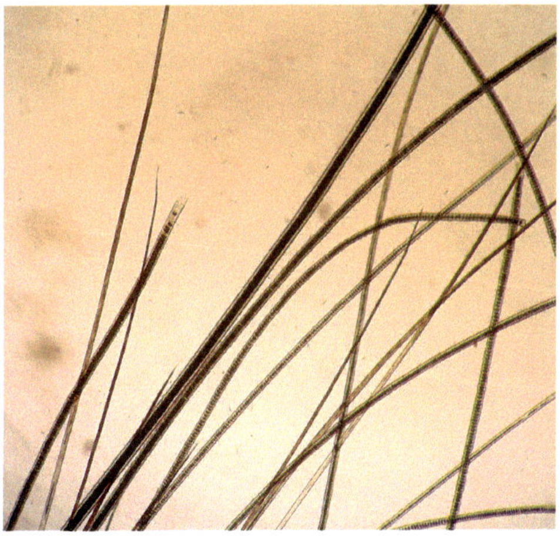

Figure 45.5. Broken hair tips.

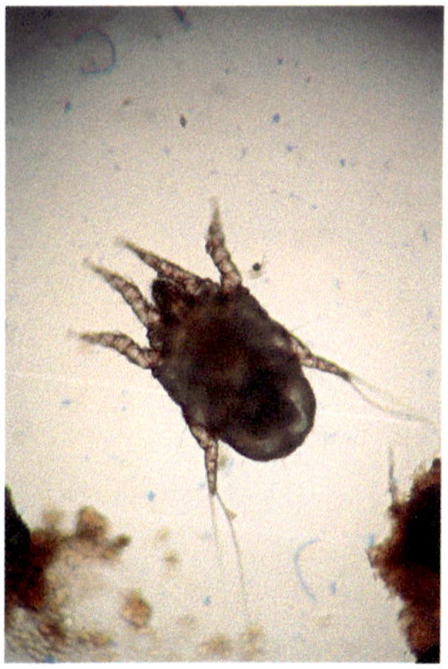

Figure 45.6. Microscopic image of *Octodectes*.

Observations

Otodectes cynotis is a primary cause of otitis externa in dogs and cats. Otitis is mainly due to a hypersensitivity reaction to the mite and is independent of the number of parasites. In many cases, parasitation by this mite does not produce clinical signs. *O. cynotis* can cause facial pruritus and self-induced alopecia in cats. Fracture of the diaphysis of the hair and the absence of some tips in the trichogram are indicative of excessive grooming caused by pruritus. The change in hair colour from black to red in cats and dogs may be due to excess saliva or tears.

Case 46

Case presentation

A spayed American Staffordshire Terrier bitch of 6 years of age was brought for consultation with chronic otitis. The dog had atopic dermatitis that was being controlled with oral oclacitinib and antiseptic baths. However, the ear problem persisted, despite treatment with different types of ear drops.

The appearance of the pinna and ear canal on examination is shown in Figures 46.1 and 46.2.

Questions

1. What type of otitis is observed in this image?
2. What secondary/perpetuating factors are complicating the otitis?
3. What treatment would be appropriate?

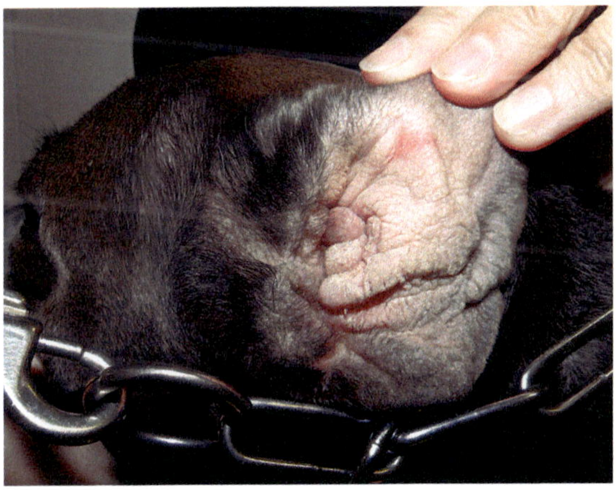

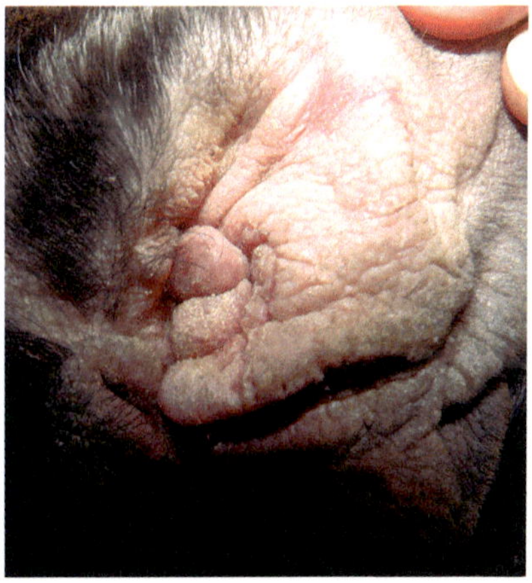

Figures 46.1 and 46.2. Appearance of the pinna and the entrance of the ear canal.

Answers Case 46

1 What type of otitis is observed in this image?

The dog has chronic erythematous and seborrhoeic otitis externa, the primary cause of which may be atopic dermatitis.

2 What secondary/perpetuating factors are complicating the otitis?

Seborrhoeic otitis is usually complicated by *Malassezia* spp. or bacterial overgrowth. In this case, cytology revealed *Malassezia* overgrowth (Fig. 46.3).

The patient's infection is a secondary process, but it is complicating the picture and exacerbating the pruritus. In addition, the ear canal is severely stenosed, contributing to the chronification of the otitis externa. Heat, humidity, and a lack of aeration favour the overgrowth of *Malassezia*. It is important to try to reverse the stenosis. If this is not possible, this patient is a strong candidate for surgical treatment.

3 What treatment would be appropriate?

Currently, oral glucocorticoid treatment at high doses for 3 or 4 weeks is recommended to reverse the process. Decreasing the inflammation will help resolve the secondary infections and pruritus.

After 3 weeks of treatment with oral corticosteroids, the pruritus and *Malassezia* overgrowth had disappeared and the stenosis of the ear canal had improved markedly (Fig. 46.4).

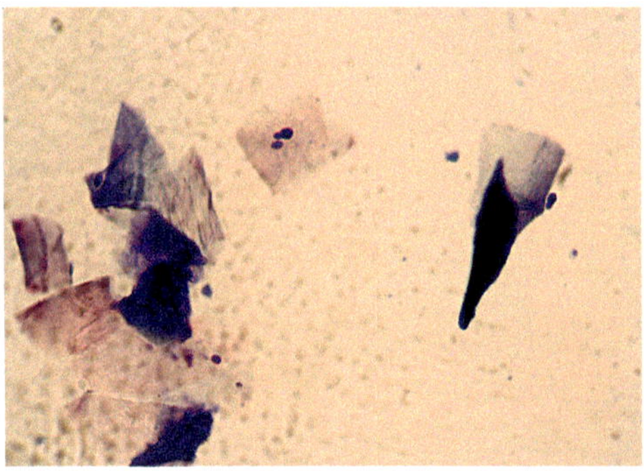

Figure 46.3. Microscopic image of the seborrhoeic exudate. Note the corneocytes, to which *Malassezia* spp. is adhered.

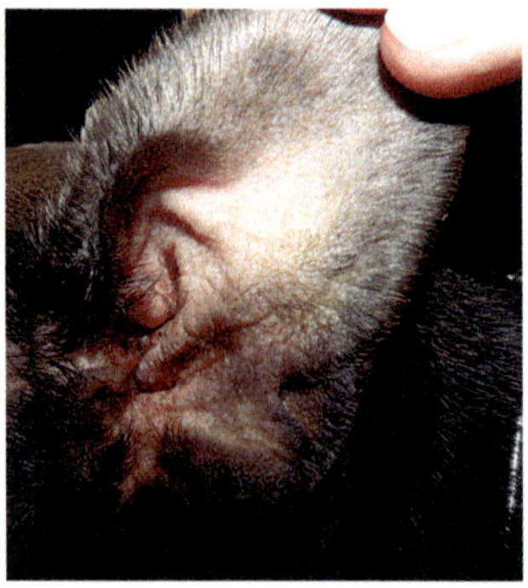

Figure 46.4. Appearance of the pinna and the entrance of the ear canal after 3 weeks of treatment with oral glucocorticoids.

Case 47

Case presentation

A 10-year-old Chow Chow bitch had been losing hair from her nose for 2 months, and then abruptly developed very painful lesions. Examination revealed a good general condition. Alopecia, erythema, exudation, and haemorrhagic crusts were observed on the nasal bridge (Fig. 47.1). The lesions were painful and did not affect the muzzle. Cytology revealed a non-septic purulent exudate.

Questions

1 What process is suggested by the types of lesions and their distribution?

2 Are there any environmental factors that could be associated with the appearance of this type of lesion?

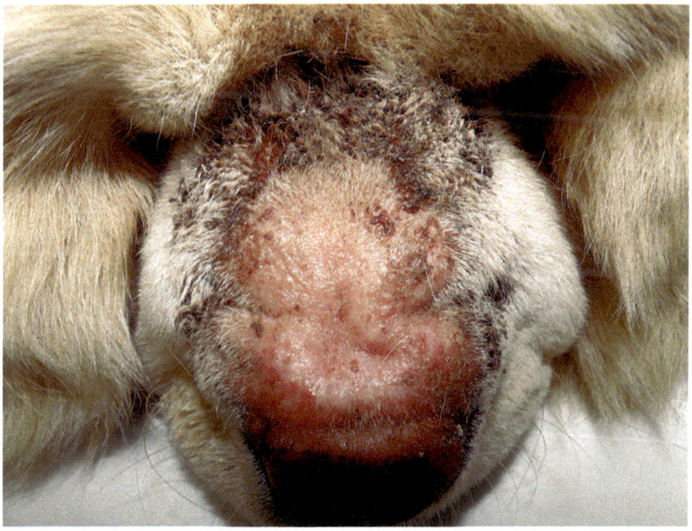

Figure 47.1. Alopecia, erythema, and crusts on the bridge of the nose.

Answers Case 47

1 What process is suggested by the types of lesions and their distribution?

In dogs with exudative lesions and alopecia of the nasal bridge, the following probable diagnoses should be considered:

- Nasal pyoderma.
- Eosinophilic folliculitis.
- Dermatophytosis.
- Leishmaniasis.
- Pemphigus foliaceus.

In this case the muzzle was unaffected, suggesting that an autoimmune disease is unlikely. Bacterial and dermatophyte cultures and a skin biopsy were performed. *Staphylococcus pseudintermedius* sensitive to beta-lactam antibiotics was detected in the bacterial culture. The biopsy revealed a neutrophilic inflammatory infiltrate with structural changes in the collagen and basophilic degeneration of the elastin. The profile was compatible with nasal pyoderma and solar dermatitis. The dermatophyte culture was negative.

2 Are there any environmental factors that could be associated with the appearance of this type of lesion?

Solar dermatitis affects areas of hairless skin such as the nose and trunk. In chronic cases preneoplastic lesions may develop (actinic keratosis, squamous cell carcinoma *in situ*). Solar dermatitis of the nose is uncommon, and its incidence is higher in dogs that live outdoors.

Figure 47.2 shows the appearance of the nasal bridge of the bitch after 1 month of antibiotic treatment and avoidance of direct solar radiation between 10:00 and 16:00 hours. If it is inevitable that the animal will be exposed to the sun, sunscreen with a protection factor of at least 30 should be applied.

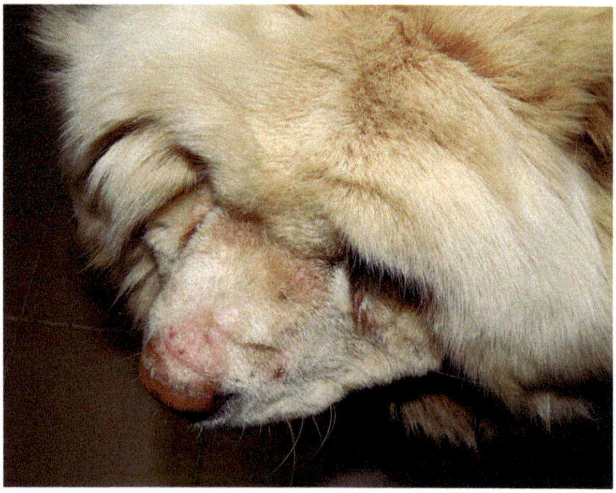

Figure 47.2. Appearance of the lesions after 3 weeks of antibiotic treatment and avoidance of sun exposure.

Case 48

Case presentation

A 3-year-old, male domestic shorthair cat was brought to the clinic by his owners, who had noticed black spots on his chin. They mentioned that they had recently adopted another kitten. Figure 48.1 shows the appearance of the chin and Figure 48.2 shows the trichogram of hair from the affected area.

Questions

1. What are this cat's lesions?
2. Could his new housemate have something to do with this condition?

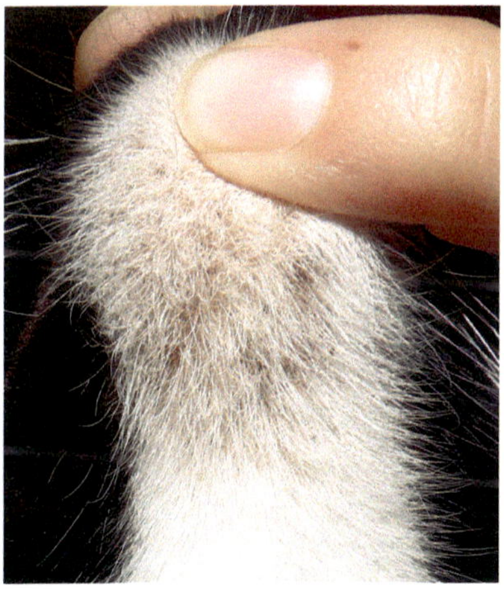

Figure 48.1. Appearance of the cat's chin.

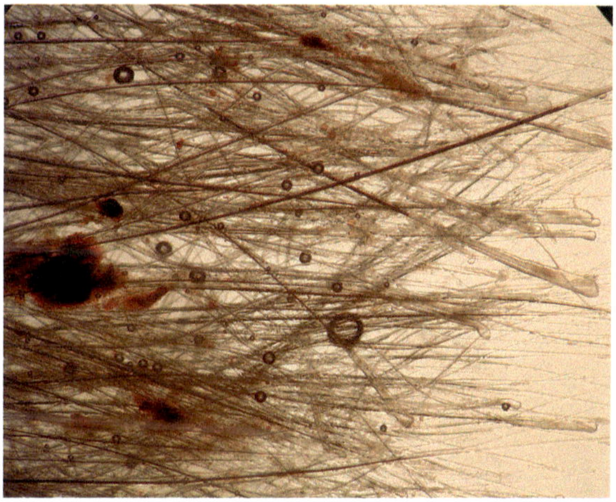

Figure 48.2. Trichogram.

Answers Case 48

1 What are this cat's lesions?

These lesions are comedones. These are follicles containing keratin debris, and appear as black spots. Commonly known as "feline acne", this is a follicular keratinisation disorder associated with glandular hyperplasia. It can also affect the upper and lower lips. In the trichogram, keratin debris is observed between the diaphyses.

The differential diagnosis should include processes such as demodicosis, dermatophytosis, *Malassezia* dermatitis, and eosinophilic granuloma.

2 Could his new housemate have something to do with this condition?

The glands in the chin area of cats produce pheromones. Cats rub their chins to mark their territory when other cats appear in their habitat. This likely accounts for the formation of comedones in this location. This is an aesthetic problem and treatment is not recommended, unless it becomes complicated by a bacterial infection resulting in folliculitis-furunculosis of the chin, which is characterised by the presence of painful papules or pustules and purulent or haemorrhagic exudate (Fig. 48.3). Topical or parenteral antibiotics should be administered if the condition becomes complicated by a secondary bacterial infection. In some cases oral prednisolone treatment may be required to prevent fibrosis and the appearance of scar tissue in the area.

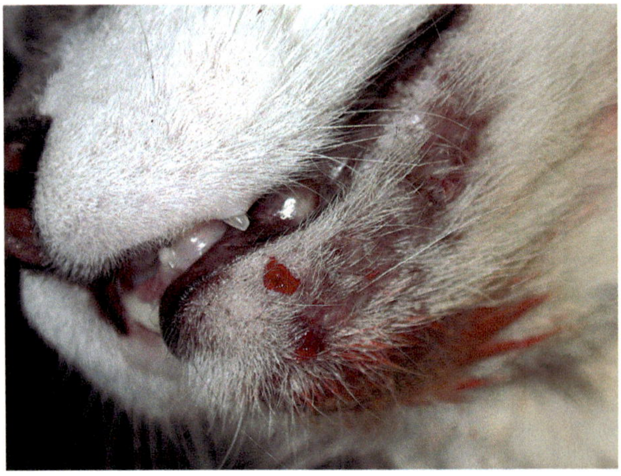

Figure 48.3. Folliculitis furunculosis of the chin secondary to acne in a cat.

Case 49

Case presentation

A male purebred Andalusian dressage horse, aged 5 years, was referred to the university veterinary hospital with cutaneous hypersensitivity in the auricular area that had appeared 3 months earlier.

On examination, greyish-white nodular and verrucous lesions, with a concave appearance and smooth surface, were observed inside both pinnae (Figs. 49.1 and 49.2).

Questions

1. With which pathology are these lesions associated in horses?
2. What topical treatment would be proposed in this case?

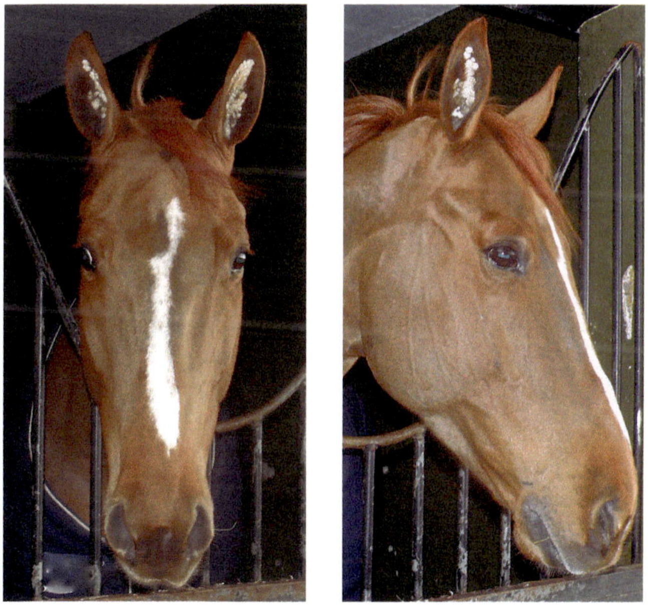

Figures 49.1 and 49.2. Verrucous-looking lesions on the inner aspect of the pinnae of a horse.

Answers Case 49

1 With which pathology are these lesions associated in horses?

These lesions are compatible with aural plaques. Aural plaque is a relatively common process that affects adult equids. This lesion is caused by a virus of the *Papillomaviridae* family that is transmitted by black flies (*Simulium* spp.).

Patients are not usually clinically affected; these lesions constitute an aesthetic problem. However, in some cases they may cause hypersensitivity of the auricular region and associated behavioural changes.

Diagnosis is established based on the clinical characteristics of the lesions. Histological confirmation is based on the presence of hyperkeratosis, parakeratosis, hyperplasia, and hexagonal intranuclear inclusions of 38–45 nm, characteristics compatible with papillomavirus infection.

2 What topical treatment would be proposed in this case?

The use of imiquimod for the treatment of equine aural plaque has been recently reported. Imiquimod is a synthetic imidazoline that modifies the immune response, and has antiviral and antitumour effects. These effects are due to the activation of Toll-like receptors, which induce the secretion from macrophages of cytokines such as interferon α (IFN-α), interleukin (IL-12), and tumour necrosis factor (TNFα). The local inflammatory response provokes a cellular immune response, which has proven effective in the treatment of pathologies such as viral papillomatosis and equine sarcoid. Dose and frequency of administration are based on the extent of the inflammatory response, which can be marked in certain cases (Fig. 49.3).

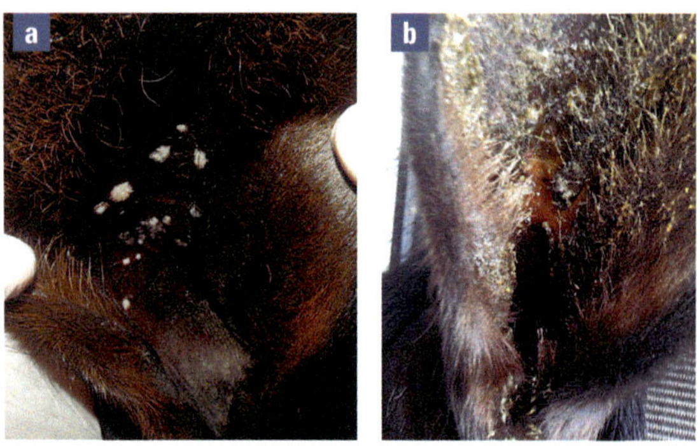

Figure 49.3. Aural plaque on the pinna of a horse (a) and appearance of the ear after treatment with imiquimod (b). An intense inflammatory reaction is observed.

Case 50

Case presentation

A 2-year-old, intact male Bull Terrier was brought for consultation with pruritus and skin lesions that secreted pus. Two months earlier he had attended a dog show, where chalk had been used to whiten his haircoat. Subsequently, the lesions appeared.

Moderate enlargement of all palpable lymph nodes was observed in the general examination. In the dermatological examination, nodular lesions with haemorrhagic exudate were observed on the head, muzzle, hocks, dorsal aspect of the tail, anus, and interdigital space (Figs. 50.1–50.4). Papular-crusted lesions were also observed on the skin of the abdomen and trunk.

Questions

1 What are the main differential diagnoses for this patient's clinical signs?

2 What diagnostic tests would be indicated?

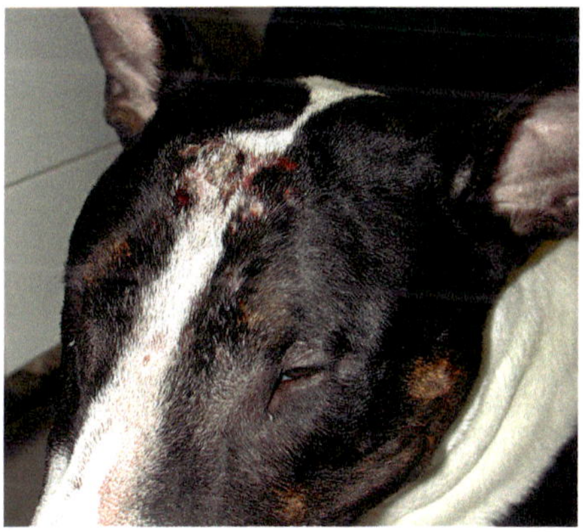

Figure 50.1. Nodular lesions with exudation and crusts on the patient's head.

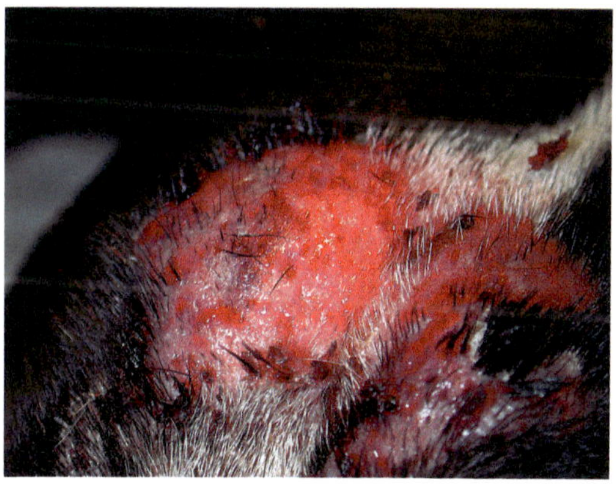

Figure 50.2. Detail of the lesions after clipping of the hair.

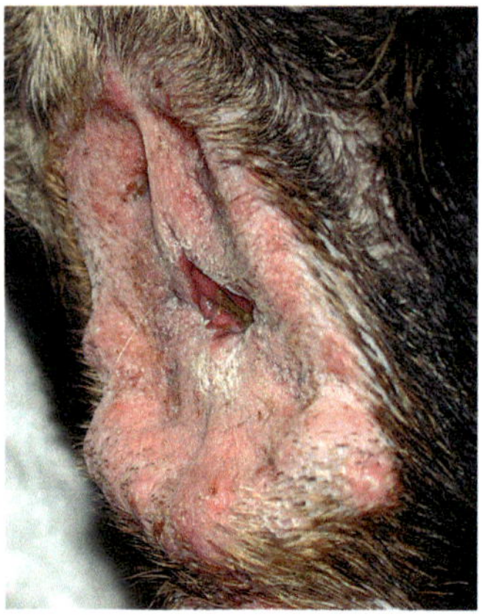

Figure 50.3. Nodules and erythema in the anal area.

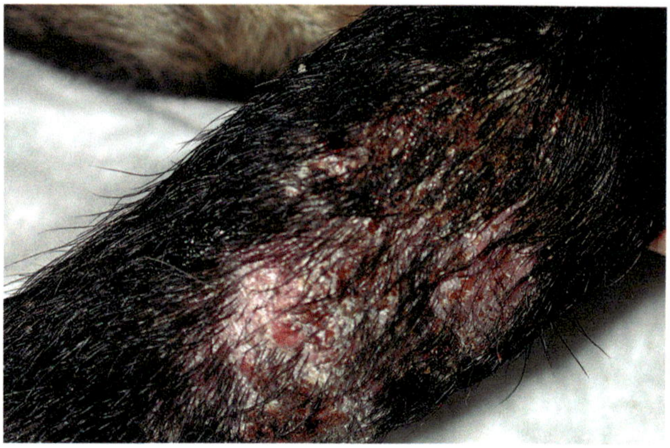

Figure 50.4. Erythema, crusts, and scaling on the dorsal aspect of the tail.

Answers Case 50

1 What are the main differential diagnoses for this patient's clinical signs?

Nodular lesions with haemorrhagic exudate are characteristic of a deep pyoderma. In this case, based on the animal's young age and clinical history, the following are the most likely differential diagnoses:

- Traumatic folliculitis-furunculosis.
- Generalised juvenile demodectic mange.
- Deep pyoderma secondary to a systemic infectious disease such as leishmaniasis.

2 What diagnostic tests would be indicated?

For this type of skin lesion, scraping, a trichogram, and cytology of the haemorrhagic exudate would be indicated. In cases involving systemic clinical signs, such as enlarged lymph nodes, cytology of the lymph node aspirate and a blood test with serology for infectious diseases compatible with the clinical signs would be indicated.

The trichogram and deep skin scraping were negative for parasites. Cytology of the haemorrhagic exudate revealed the presence of polymorphonuclear neutrophils, eosinophils, and macrophages, and degenerative changes in neutrophils in which microorganisms (cocci) were evident. Lymph node cytology was compatible with reactive lymph node hyperplasia. The results of the blood and urine tests were within the range of normality, except for mild hypergammaglobulinaemia. Tests for the presence of antibodies against *Leishmania* and *Ehrlichia* were negative.

Given the severity of the clinical picture, culture and antibiogram of the exudate were performed, as well as a lesion biopsy. While awaiting the results, treatment with oral cephalexin at 22 mg/kg every 12 hours was initiated.

Histology showed an intense purulent inflammatory response around the hair follicles with ruptured follicles and foreign body reaction (Figs. 50.5 and 50.6). *Staphylococcus aureus* that was resistant to the majority of antibiotics tested, except for rifampicin, grew in the bacterial culture. Based on this finding, oral rifampicin was administered for 6 weeks, with good response (Fig. 50.7).

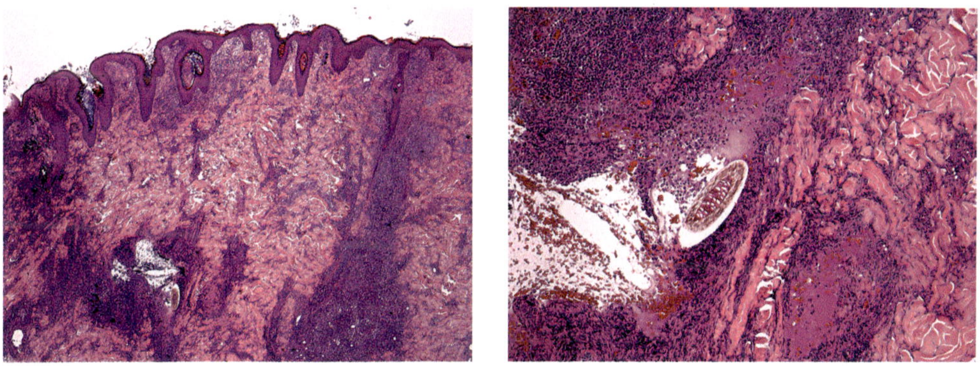

Figures 50.5 and 50.6. Histological images showing an intense inflammatory exudate around the hair follicles and rupture of the follicles (furunculosis).

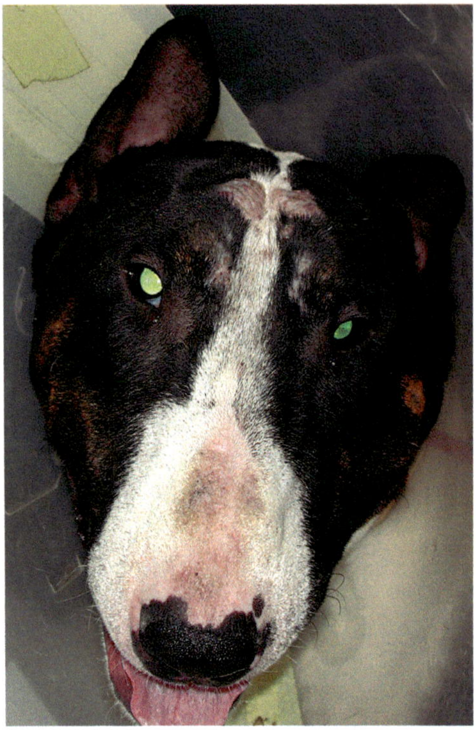

Figure 50.7. Appearance of the patient after 6 weeks of treatment with the appropriate antibiotic.

Observations

Traumatic folliculitis occurs secondary to an aggression affecting the hair follicle (aggressive washing or brushing, topical treatments, activities that macerate, irritate, or apply pressure to a certain area). This inflammatory process occurs with secondary bacterial infections. Due to the intense inflammatory process, folliculitis evolves to furunculosis; the keratin debris is treated as a foreign body, giving rise to local pyogranulomatous reactions.

S. aureus is a bacterium that is a component of the skin microbiota of humans. In this case, the owner of the dog was being treated for viral hepatitis. Immunosuppressed people or animals, who are undergoing chronic antibiotic therapy or who have been hospitalised, are more likely to be carriers of multiresistant bacteria and can be a source of contagion for people or animals with which they are in contact.

Case 51

Case presentation

A 10-year-old, intact male Yorkshire Terrier was brought to the dermatology clinic by his owners, who reported that he begun licking his body and legs over 1 year earlier, and was very restless. They had also noticed that the dog smelled badly. His general condition was good, but he had lost weight. He had been treated with corticosteroids and oclacitinib, but regurgitated the medication. The condition responded partially to injectable glucocorticoids. A previous urine infection had been treated with antibiotics. Almost 1 year before the consultation he had undergone basic biochemical analyses and an ultrasound, the results of which were normal. He was fed on a commercial salmon-based diet and lived with another dog that was healthy. The owners themselves had not been affected by any lesions. The family often travelled to the coast (Valencia, Spain).

The results of the general examination were normal. In the dermatological examination it was observed that the hair of the trunk had become matted due to intense oily seborrhoea (Figs. 51.1 and 51.2). Mild interdigital erythema was also observed.

Questions

1. To which disease characterised by oily seborrhoea are Terriers predisposed?
2. What could be the cause of the bad odour?

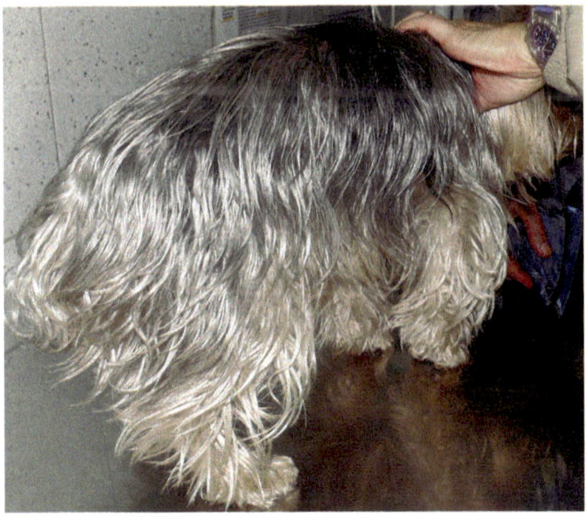

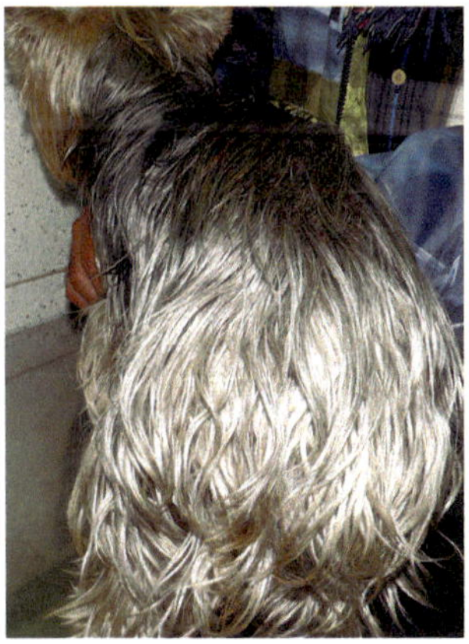

Figures 51.1 and 51.2. Oily seborrhoea that affects the trunk. Note the matted hair.

Answers Case 51

1 To which disease characterised by oily seborrhoea are Terriers predisposed?

The Yorkshire Terrier, West Highland White Terrier, and Shih Tzu breeds are predisposed to seborrhoeic dermatitis associated with the proliferation of *Demodex injai*.

D. injai was first described in 1990 and is a long-lived mite that lives in the hair follicle and sebaceous glands and ducts (Fig. 51.3). It causes a form of demodicosis that differs clinically to that caused by *Demodex canis*, and is generally characterised by oily seborrhoea, especially on the face and upper line of the body. Since the number of mites tends to be small, hair loss is mild.

2 What could be the cause of the bad odour?

The bad odour in this dog could be due to secondary infections (bacterial, *Malassezia)* or to the seborrhoea itself.

In this case, multiple skin scrapings were performed, analysis of which revealed a small number of *D. injai* mites (Fig. 51.3). Skin surface cytology showed bacterial and *Malassezia* spp. overgrowth.

The patient was treated with oral fluralaner and antiseptic baths, and showed a good response to treatment.

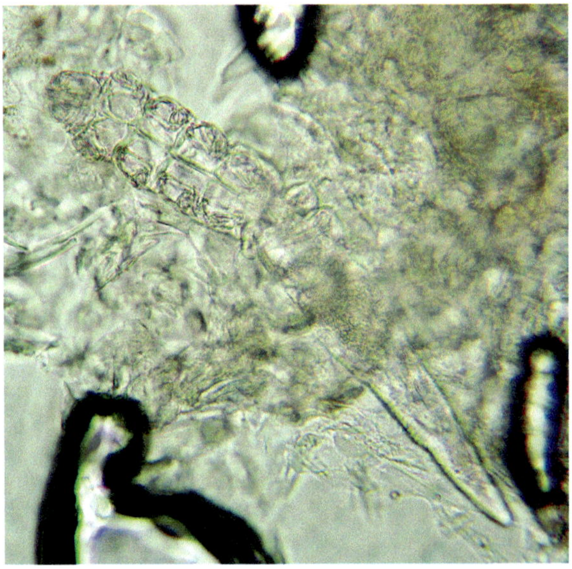

Figure 51.3. *Demodex injai.*

Case 52

Case presentation

A 7-month-old male mongrel dog developed a pruritic condition affecting the trunk area. His general condition was good. He had spent a few days in a village 3 weeks earlier. He did not live with other animals and the owners had no lesions. On examination, erythema and crusted papular lesions were observed on the back and the extremities. The mites shown in Figure 52.1 were detected in the skin scraping.

Questions

1. What parasite is this?
2. What treatment would be appropriate?

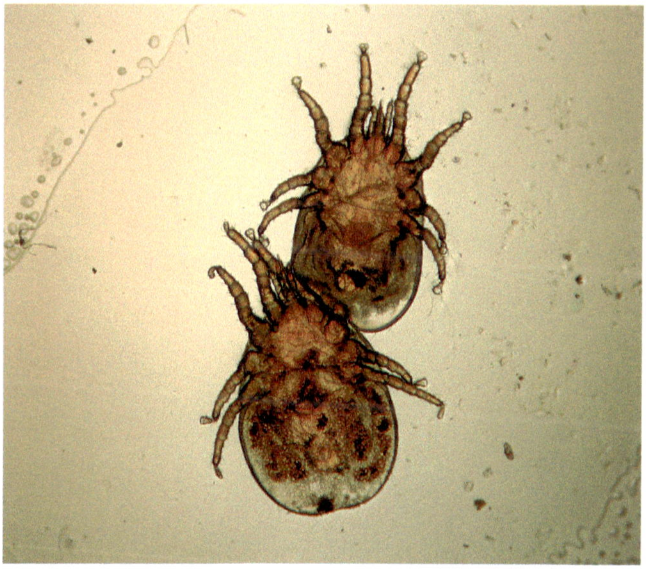

Figure 52.1. External mite.

Answers Case 52

1 What parasite is this?

This is the *Dermanyssus gallinae* mite. This parasite affects poultry, wild and caged birds, dogs, cats, and humans. This mite lives in nests and in crevices in cages and houses. This rare parasite is found in pets that have access to poultry houses and causes an inflammatory reaction, predominantly affecting the back and extremities.

2 What treatment would be appropriate?

D. gallinae responds to general acaricides, in solution, aerosol, and pipette formulations.

Case 53

Case presentation

A 2-year-old, intact male Australian Shepherd had an eyelid lesion that appeared 6 months earlier and had since progressively increased in size. The appearance of the lesion was followed by spots on the ears and loss of the nails. The dog was in good general health and appeared to be unaffected by the skin lesions, but did lick his legs. His diet consisted of medium-grade dog food. He lived in a house in Madrid, with other dogs that had no skin lesions. None of the people who shared the apartment with the dog had any skin lesions. The dog received antiparasitic treatment in the form of permethrin (pipettes) during the summer and an insecticide collar. Analysis of a skin scraping had proved negative for leishmaniasis.

The results of the general examination were normal, except for moderate lymphadenopathy. In the dermatological examination, alopecia with hyperpigmentation, scaling, and mild exudation was observed on the eyelid, the inner aspect of the pinna, and the distal portion of the forelimbs (Figs. 53.1 and 53.2). The dog exhibited generalised onychodystrophy and onychorrhexis (Fig. 53.3), and showed pain during the nail examination.

Brushing and a subsequent trichogram revealed no parasites or fungal spores. Small numbers of neutrophils and melanophages were observed in the exudate cytology. Bacterial overgrowth was detected in the nail sample.

Questions

1. Is this dog's multifocal alopecia inflammatory or noninflammatory?
2. Based on the alopecia and nail lesions, what are the relevant differential diagnoses?
3. What would be the diagnostic test of choice?

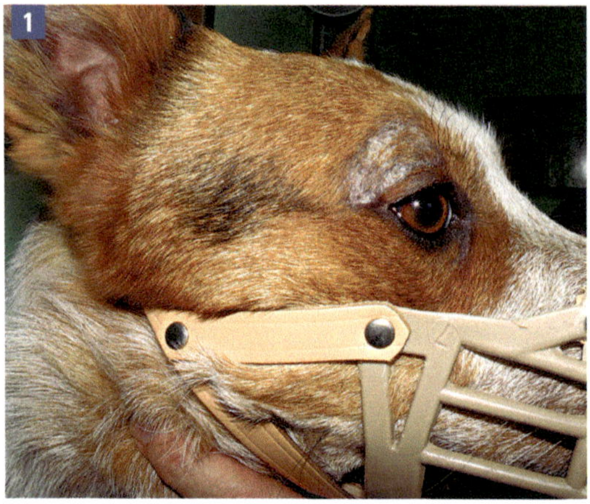

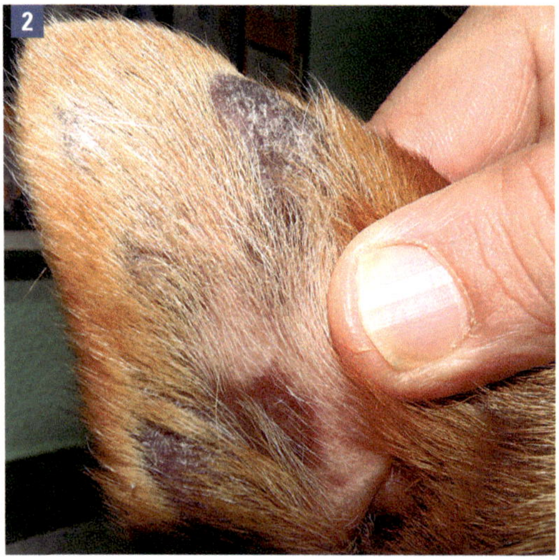

Figures 53.1 and 53.2. Multifocal alopecia with scaling and hyperpigmentation on the eyelid and the inner aspect of the pinna.

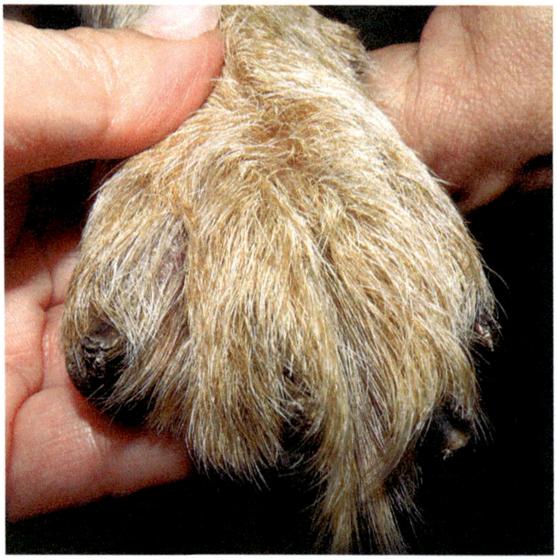

Figure 53.3. Onychodystrophy and onychorrhexis. Note the abnormal direction of nail growth.

Answers Case 53

1 Is this dog's multifocal alopecia inflammatory or noninflammatory?

This patient's alopecia appears to be inflammatory and multifocal, since exudation and inflammatory cells are evident.

2 Based on the alopecia and nail lesions, what are the relevant differential diagnoses?

The following are the most likely differential diagnoses of inflammatory multifocal alopecia:

- Dermatophytosis.
- Demodicosis.
- Bacterial folliculitis.
- Leishmaniasis.
- Alopecia areata.
- Sebaceous adenitis.
- Vasculitis.
- Ischaemic dermatopathies.
- Pemphigus foliaceus.
- Epitheliotropic lymphoma.

Given the presence of onychodystrophy and onychorrhexis, the following should also be included:

- Bacterial infections.
- Onychomycosis.
- Lupoid onychodystrophy.
- Vasculitis.
- Ischaemic dermatopathies.

3 What would be the diagnostic test of choice?

Given the multifocal inflammatory alopecia and nail dystrophy, and the patient's age and breed, the most probable diagnosis is a vascular problem. To identify the cause, a skin biopsy was recommended.

Histology was compatible with a vascular lesion, with only a mild inflammatory process observed. Ischaemic dermatopathy/cell-poor vasculitis affects the dermal collagen and hair follicles, and has several forms. Juvenile ischaemic dermatopathy is a hereditary disease to which several breeds, including the Australian Shepherd, are predisposed. It is characterised by alopecia on the face, pinnae, bony prominences, digits, and tail. The nails may be dystrophic and exhibit onychorrhexis and onychomadesis.

The patient was treated with cyclosporine, oral pentoxifylline, and fatty acid supplements. Three months after treatment, the alopecic lesions had almost completely resolved and the periungual inflammation had improved, although the onychodystrophy persisted (Figs. 53.4 and 53.5).

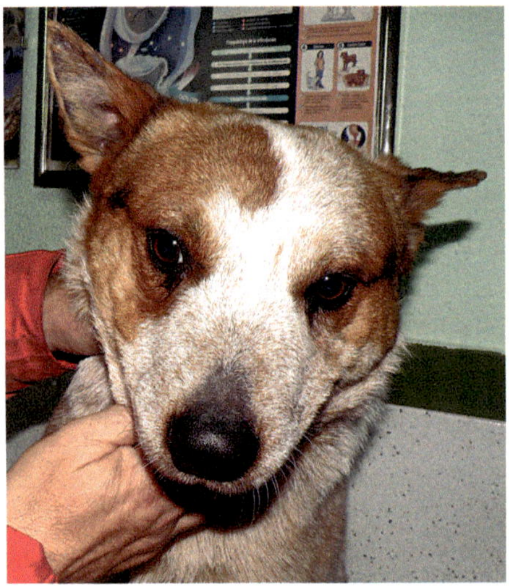

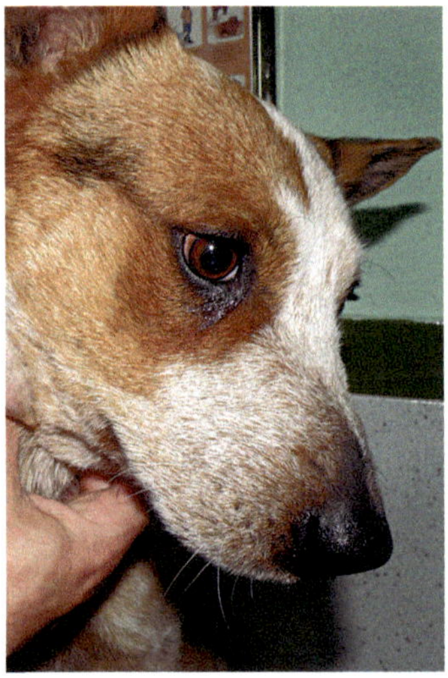

Figures 53.4 and 53.5. Appearance of the dog after 3 months of treatment with oral cyclosporine and pentoxifylline. The alopecia of the eyelid has resolved, although some alopecia and hyperpigmentation on the inner aspect of the pinna persists.

Case 54

Case presentation

An intact male Yorkshire Terrier of 9 years of age was brought to the clinic with a lump that had ruptured. Beginning 9 months earlier, he had developed several "lumps" that remained the same size, or grew and ultimately ruptured. At the moment of the consultation he had a large lump on his back that appeared to irritate him.

Examination revealed the presence of numerous subcutaneous, non-painful nodules and tumours (Figs. 54.1–54.3). In one of the nodules on the back was an open pore containing a keratin plug that caused pain when palpated (Fig. 54.4). Images of the cytology of the pore content are shown in Figures 54.5 and 54.6.

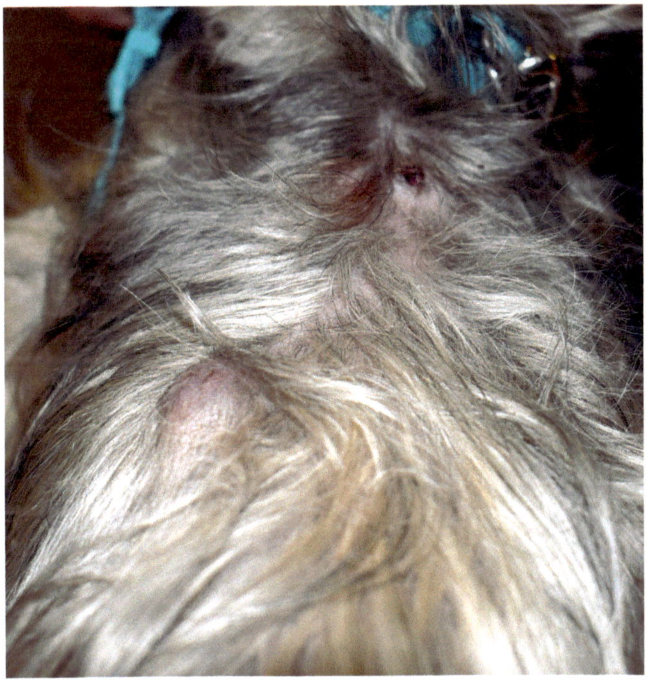

Figure 54.1. Appearance of the dorsal area of the patient; two nodules are visible, one of which contains an open pore.

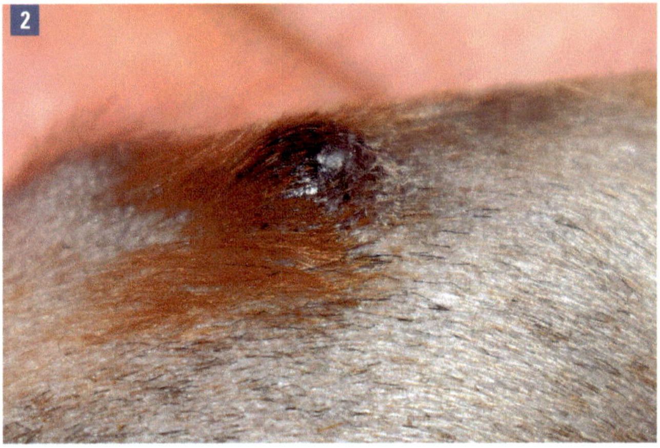

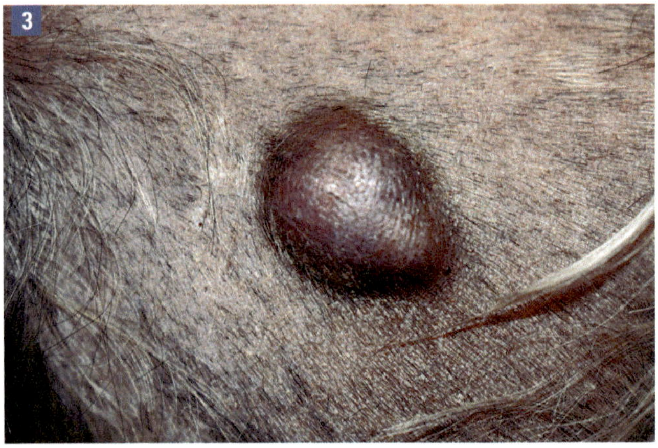

Figures 54.2 and 54.3. Nodules distributed across the trunk of the patient. The hair has been clipped to allow better visualisation of the lesions.

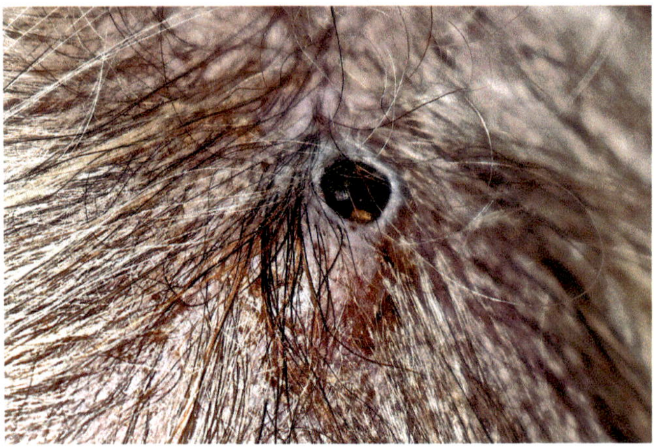

Figure 54.4. Detail of the open pore with a keratin plug.

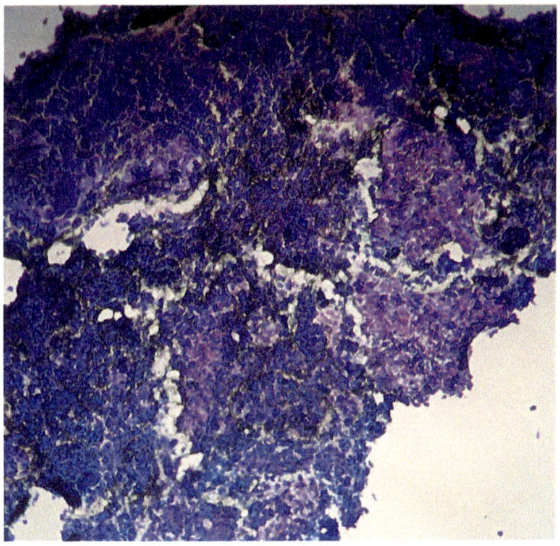

Figure 54.5. Low-magnification image showing cytology of the aspirated material.

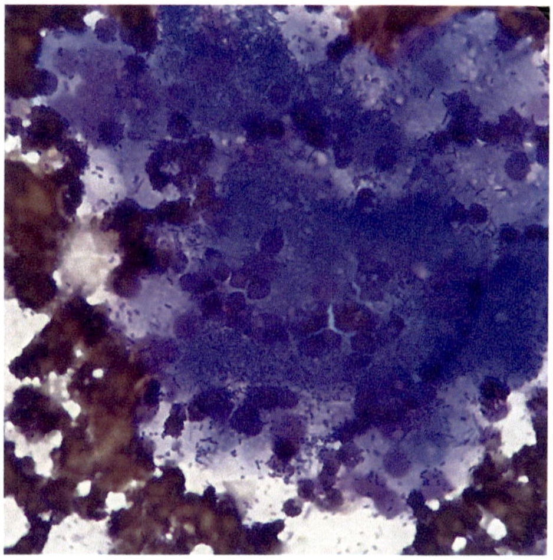

Figure 54.6. High-magnification image showing cytology of the aspirated material.

Questions

1 What type of tumour does this dog most likely have?

2 What is observed in the nodule cytology?

Answers Case 54

1 What type of tumour does this dog most likely have?

The appearance of the tumours and their clinical characteristics correspond to infundibular keratinising acanthoma. These are benign tumours of epithelial origin that arise from the wall of the hair follicle. They usually appear as single or multiple well-defined cutaneous or subcutaneous masses, which can be firm or fluid-filled and vary in size from 0.5 to 4 cm in diameter.

The nodules can be partially alopecic and usually contain a dilated central pore of variable size that opens to the skin surface. The pore releases brownish-grey material, which in some cases forms a hard keratin plug, resembling a horn. Some tumours are located in the deep dermis and do not open to the surface.

The average age of onset is 7 years. The Norwegian Elkhound, Lhasa Apso, Pekingese, Yorkshire Terrier, and German Shepherd breeds show a particular predisposition.

2 What is observed in the nodule cytology?

In the first, low-magnification image of the nodule cytology, abundant keratin debris and remnants of melanin are evident. Material formed by amorphous keratin with associated bacterial contamination can be seen. Anucleated keratinised epithelial cells and cholesterol crystals are also evident (Figs. 54.7 and 54.8).

Histology reveals cavities that are filled with laminated keratin and lined with stratified epithelial cells, and may contain a pore that connects to the skin surface.

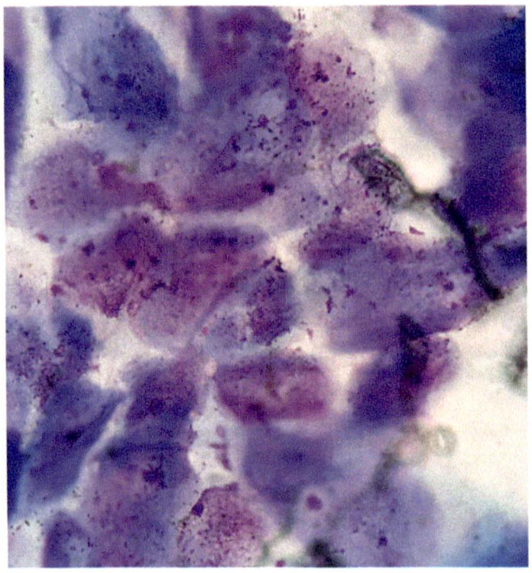

Figure 54.7. Anucleated keratinised epithelial cells typical of this type of tumour.

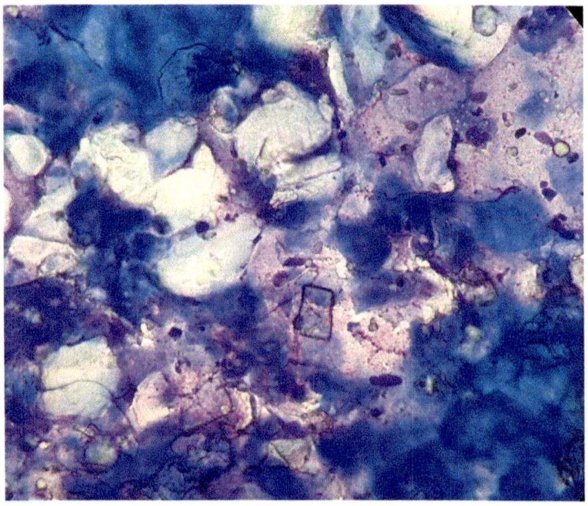

Figure 54.8. Cholesterol crystals and amorphous keratinised material in a case of infundibular keratinising acanthoma.

Observations

Infundibular keratinising adenomas may be difficult to differentiate clinically from non-tumoural epidermal cysts.

Surgical resection is the treatment of choice. In cases involving multiple adenomas, treatment with topical imiquimod or oral retinoid derivatives has been proposed.

Case 55

Case presentation

The patient was a 7-year-old, spayed, female domestic shorthair cat with anorexia, which had begun 2 days earlier and resulted in weight loss. The cat had been receiving oral ketoconazole and topical clotrimazole for the previous 15 days for treatment of a possible dermatophytosis associated with the appearance of hairless patches. She also had asthma, which was diagnosed at 2 years of age and had been treated continuously with oral prednisolone at 2 mg/day. The cat continuously licked her entire body.

In the general examination the animal appeared dejected and showed pain during examination of the abdomen. Hypotrichosis and diffuse alopecia were evident around the neck and on the skin of the abdomen (Figs. 55.1 and 55.2). Apart from alopecia, no other skin lesions were observed. A radiographic study of the thoracic cavity revealed a chronic bronchial pattern. Abdominal ultrasound showed a focal peritoneal reaction in the area of the hepatic hilum that was suggestive of pancreatitis. The urinary bladder contained non-mineral sediment in suspension. Blood and urine tests confirmed pancreatitis and bacterial cystitis. No parasites or fungal spores were observed in the examination of the hair of the affected areas. The appearance of the tips of the hair shafts is shown in Figure 55.3.

Questions

1. What is suggested by the appearance of the tips of the hair shafts as observed in the trichogram?
2. What is the relationship between the patient's general clinical signs and the dermatological lesions?

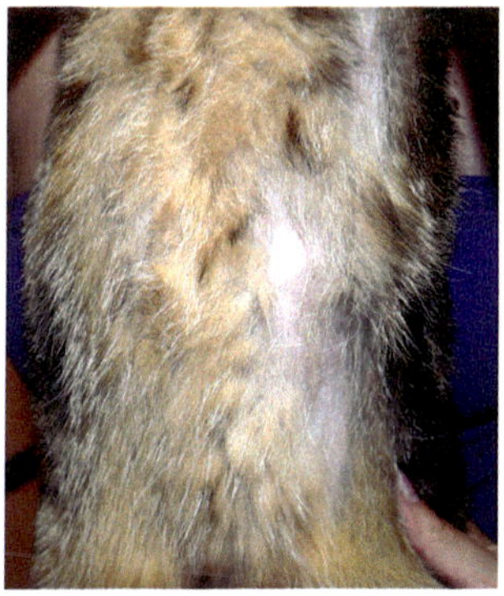
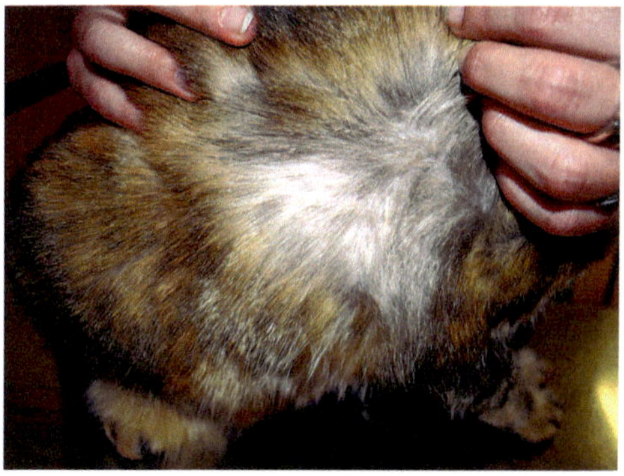

Figures 55.1 and 55.2. Alopecia and hypotrichosis on the skin of the abdomen and lateral aspect of the neck.

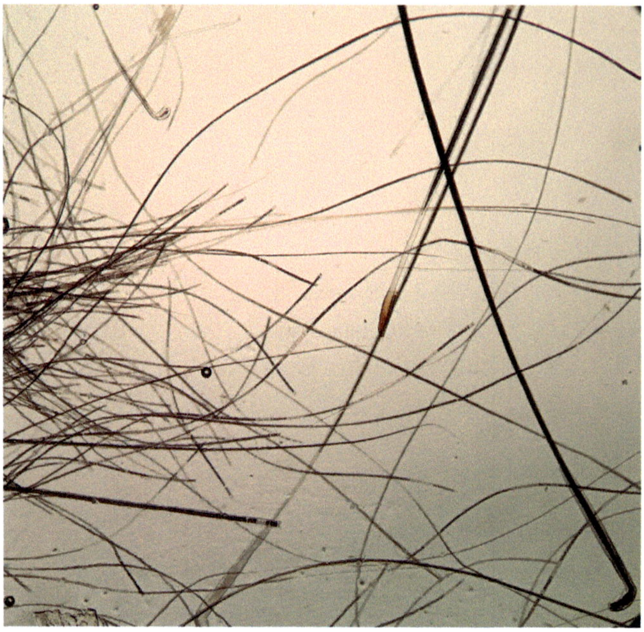

Figure 55.3. Appearance of hair tips in the trichogram.

Answers Case 55

1 What is suggested by the appearance of the tips of the hair shafts as observed in the trichogram?

The broken hair tips suggest that the cat's licking is the cause of the loss of hair, and that this is therefore a case of self-induced alopecia.

2 What is the relationship between the patient's general clinical signs and the dermatological lesions?

Self-induced alopecia in cats can be caused by pruritus (allergies, bacterial or fungal infections, parasites), pain (osteoarthritis, chronic inflammatory processes, etc.), or behavioural disorders (anxiety, stereotypies).

In this case, the oral ketoconazole that the patient had been receiving over the previous 15 days may have induced the anorexia and pancreatitis; this drug is contraindicated in cats on account of its adverse effects. The cystitis may be secondary to the chronic glucocorticoid administration.

Once the bacterial cystitis was resolved with antibiotic treatment, the cat stopped grooming continuously, and the hypotrichosis and alopecia resolved. The response to treatment suggests that the self-induced alopecia may have been a result of the pain and discomfort caused by the cystitis.

Case 56

Case presentation

An intact male Cocker Spaniel of 3 years of age was brought to the clinic by his owners, who reported loss of the nails over the preceding 5 months. The dog had no other skin lesions. He had undergone serology for leishmaniasis and ehrlichiosis, and had tested negative in both cases. A few months earlier he had experienced an episode of diarrhoea and haematuria. He lived with two other healthy dogs, and his owners had no skin lesions. He lived in an apartment in Madrid and had not travelled in recent months. His was fed a medium-grade diet, and he was fully vaccinated and dewormed on a monthly basis. Clinical signs had improved with antibiotic treatment.

The general examination revealed no findings of note. In the dermatological examination, exudate and crusting was observed around all nails. Abnormal growth of the nails, which had become soft and fragmented, was also evident (Figs. 56.1–56.3). The upper part of some nails broke off easily and the soft tissue of the digit appeared swollen (Fig. 56.4). The dog showed considerable pain on palpation of the nails. No other skin lesions were detected.

Cytology of the periungual exudate showed neutrophils with toxic changes and the presence of intracellular and extracellular bacteria (cocci).

Questions

1. What lesions affect the nails of this patient? What are they called?
2. What are the most likely diagnoses and what would be the diagnostic procedure of choice?

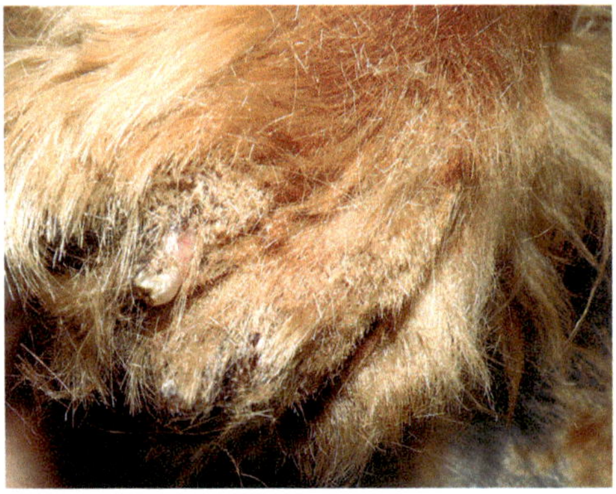

Figure 56.1. Exudate and crusting around the nails.

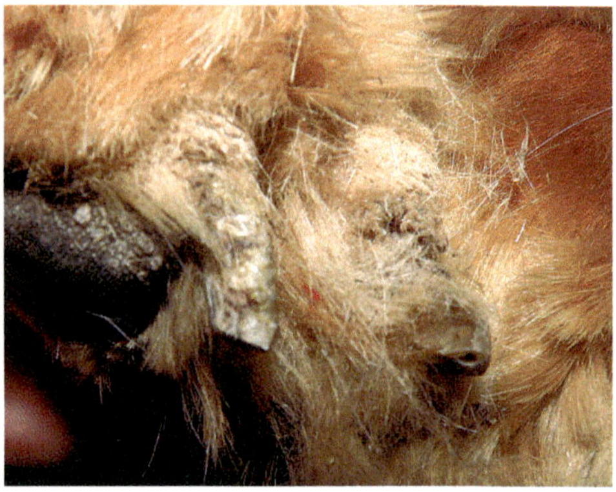

Figure 56.2. Crusts and nails displaying superficial cracking and fragmentation.

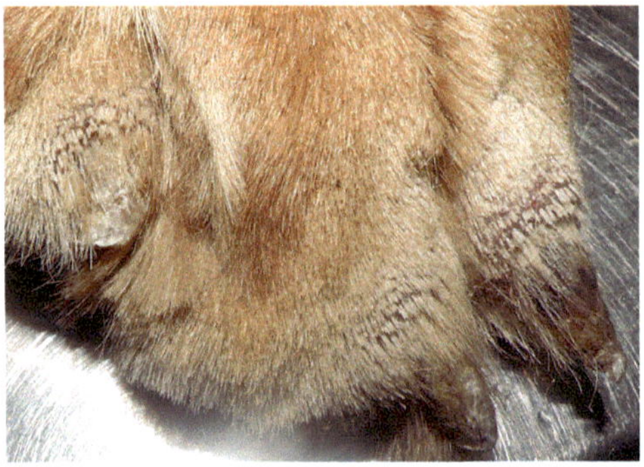

Figure 56.3. Softening of the tip of the nail.

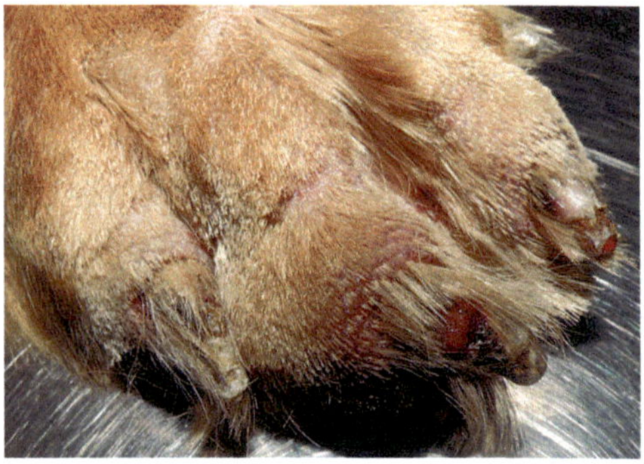

Figure 56.4. Distal separation and shedding of the nail.

Answers Case 56

1 What lesions affect the nails of this patient? What are they called?

In the nails of this dog the following pathological processes are observed:

- Paronychia: inflammation/infection in the nail fold (Fig. 56.1).
- Onychorrhexis: rupture and fissures in the nail that promote fracture (Figs. 56.2 and 56.5).
- Onychomalacia: softening of the nails (Fig. 56.3).
- Onychomadesis: shedding of the nail as a result of onycholysis; the nail detaches distally and the separation progresses proximally (Fig. 56.4).
- Onychodystrophy: abnormal formation and growth of the nail (Figs. 56.2–56.5).
- Onychalgia: pain affecting the nails.

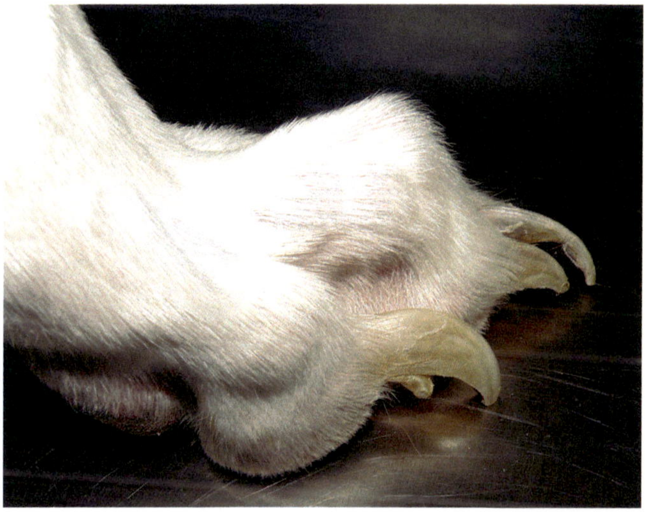

Figure 56.5. Onychorrhexis and onychodystrophy in a dog. Onychogryphosis (hypertrophy and abnormal curvature of the nails) are also evident.

2 What are the most likely diagnoses and what would be the diagnostic procedure of choice?

In the absence of other skin lesions, the differential diagnosis in dogs in which multiple nails are affected should include the following:

- Symmetric lupoid onychodystrophy.
- Vasculitis and ischaemic dermatopathies.
- Postvaccinal reactions.

In this case, no vaccinations administered in the previous 6 months were recorded in the medical record. It was decided to perform a nail biopsy. Histopathology showed a lichenoid mononuclear infiltrate. Although these findings may correspond to an inflammatory response to different diseases (adverse reaction to food and drugs, leishmaniasis), in this case the clinical picture was strongly indicative of symmetric lupoid onychodystrophy.

The dog was treated with a combination of doxycycline, nicotinamide (niacinamide in the American pharmacopoeia), pentoxifylline, vitamin E, and essential fatty acids. Four months after starting treatment, marked improvements in the paronychia and pain were observed, and the onychomadesis had disappeared. However, the onychorrhexis and onychodystrophy persisted (Fig. 56.6).

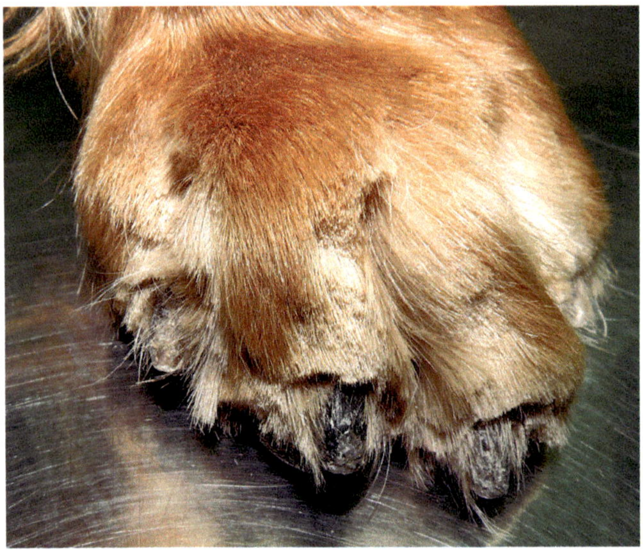

Figure 56.6. Appearance of the patient's nails after 4 months of treatment. The paronychia and onychomadesis have improved, but onychorrhexis and onychodystrophy persist.

Case 57

Case presentation

Figures 57.1 and 57.2 show the appearance of the nails and the skin of the digits of a 9-year-old Golden Retriever who had undergone 4 weeks of radiotherapy treatment for squamous cell carcinoma. The dog licked his leg and appeared to be bothered by the lesions.

Questions

1. What is the name of this pathology and what lesions are observed?
2. What treatment would be appropriate?

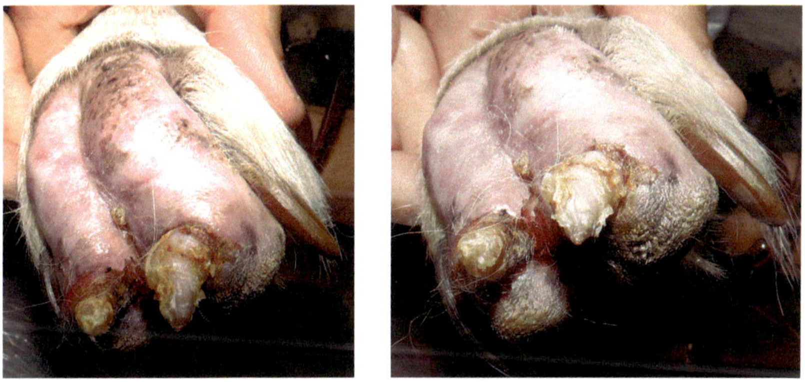

Figures 57.1 and 57.2. Appearance of the nails and the skin of the digits 4 weeks after beginning radiotherapy.

Answers Case 57

1 What is the name of this pathology and what lesions are observed?

This is a case of radiation dermatitis. The following lesions are evident: alopecia, erythema, oedema, periungual exudation, and onychodystrophy. In more severe cases, necrosis of the skin and adjacent tissues may occur. The incidence of side effects depends on the total radiation dose, dose per session, treatment time, energy, type of radiation, and exposed body area.

2 What treatment would be appropriate?

Topical corticosteroids, soothing emollients, and tissue regenerators such as dexpanthenol are used. Patients undergoing radiation therapy should avoid solar radiation. Recommended preventive measures include washing with mild soap of the area to be irradiated (to decrease the bacterial load) and the use of moisturisers and emollients such as aloe vera and creams containing sucralfate. Oral administration of pentoxifylline is also recommended.

The patient was treated with ointments containing corticosteroids, antibiotics, and emollient and moisturising agents. In this case, the hair loss turned out to be a permanent side effect (Fig. 57.3).

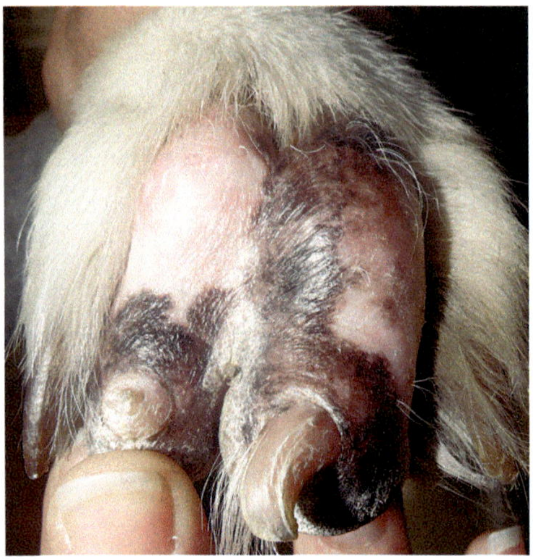

Figure 57.3. Appearance of the patient's digits after treatment with topical corticosteroids and antibiotics and emollients. The inflammation has disappeared, but the alopecia persists.

Case 58

Case presentation

A castrated male Persian cat of 9 years of age was referred to the oncology clinic with multiple melanomas on the eyelids. Examination revealed a large number of highly pigmented cysts on the upper and lower eyelids of both eyes and on the skin of the lacrimal fold of the right eye (Figs. 58.1 and 58.2).

The content of the cystic lesions was a dark coloured liquid with a granular appearance.

Questions

1. What disease does this clinical picture suggest?
2. What treatment would be appropriate?

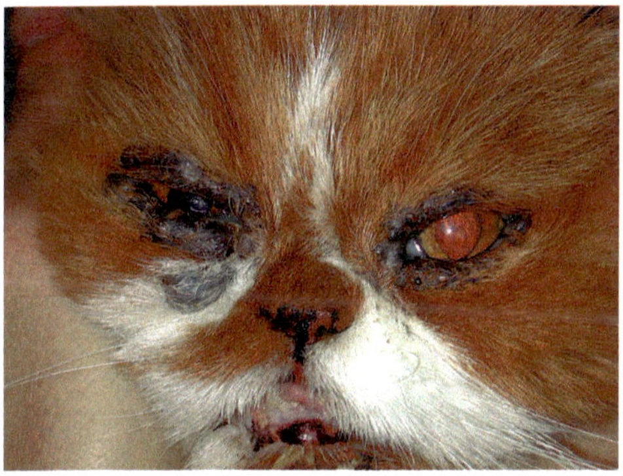

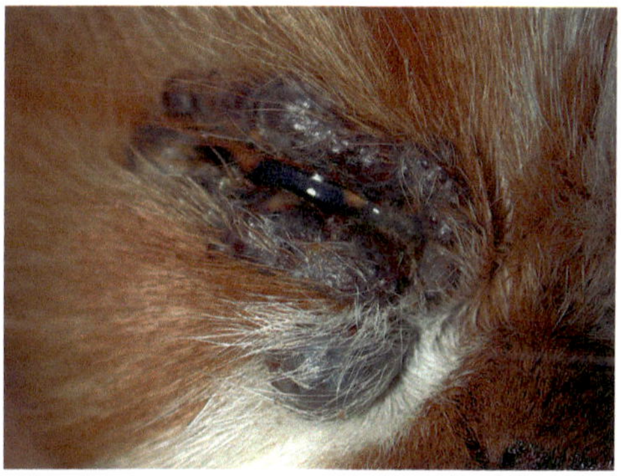

Figures 58.1 and 58.2. Nodular and hyperpigmented lesions on the patient's eyelids.

Answers Case 58

1 What disease does this clinical picture suggest?

This clinical picture is compatible with epitrichial cystadenoma or apocrine hidrocystoma. The cysts originate in the apocrine sweat glands in the palpebral skin and in the glands of Moll inside the border of the eyelid. They can appear in cats of any age, and no sexual predisposition has been reported. Cystadenomas are typically brown to black elevated cysts that develop on the periocular skin. The colour of the cystic fluid is attributed to hemosiderin and ceroid substances. Fluid aspiration can help differentiate these cysts from melanomas, but definitive diagnosis requires an excisional biopsy.

2 What treatment would be appropriate?

These cysts can be treated by surgical laser or with silver nitrate. Cytoreduction treatment with 20 % trichloroacetic acid has also been described.

Case 59

Case presentation

The patient, an intact male mongrel of 5 years of age, presented with skin lesions on the abdomen that had appeared 3 months earlier. The owners had applied povidone iodine and an antibiotic ointment, to no effect. Some lesions improved without treatment, but new lesions subsequently appeared. The lesions caused mild pruritus. The patient had been tested for leishmaniasis, with a negative result.

In the general examination, slight enlargement of the prescapular and popliteal lymph nodes was observed. Nodular skin lesions were observed on the ventral aspect of the neck, the skin of the abdomen, the prepuce, the outer aspect of the thigh, and the tail (Figs. 59.1–59.3). In some lesions an area of necrosis with central crusting and plaque formation was evident (Figs. 59.3 and 59.4).

Aspiration cytology of different nodules was performed (Figs. 59.5).

Questions

1. What type of skin pattern does this patient display, and what are the most likely diagnoses?
2. What cells are observed in the cytology and what type of pathology do they suggest?

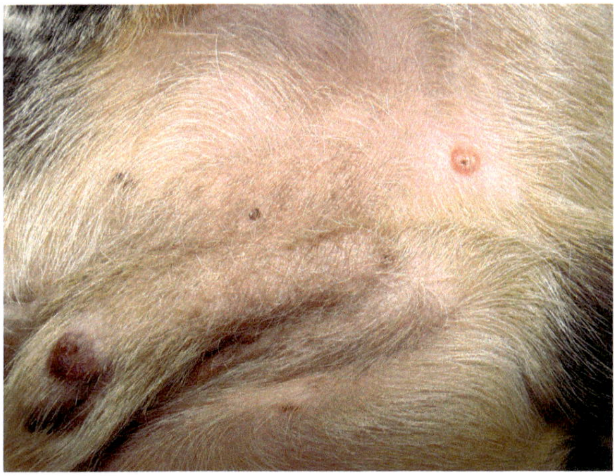

Figure 59.1. Nodular skin lesions on the abdomen and prepuce.

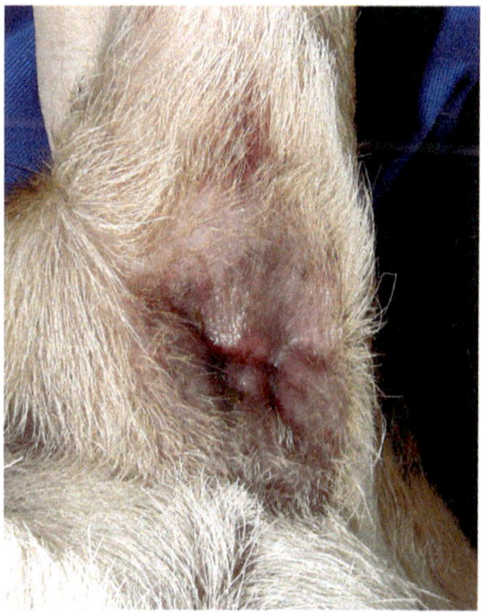

Figure 59.2. Nodular lesion at the base of the tail.

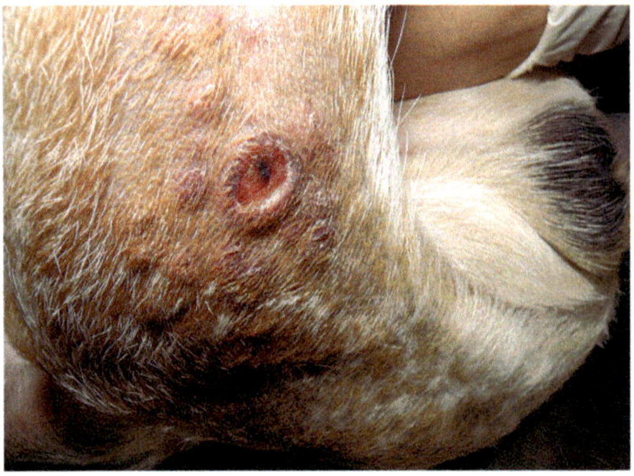

Figure 59.3. Multiple nodules on the skin of the outer aspect of the thigh. Some nodules display a zone of central necrosis, with ulceration and crusting.

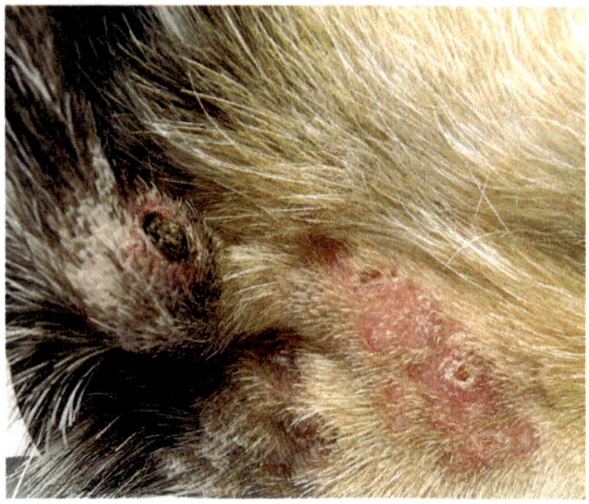

Figure 59.4. Plaque and nodule with central necrosis on the ventral aspect of the neck.

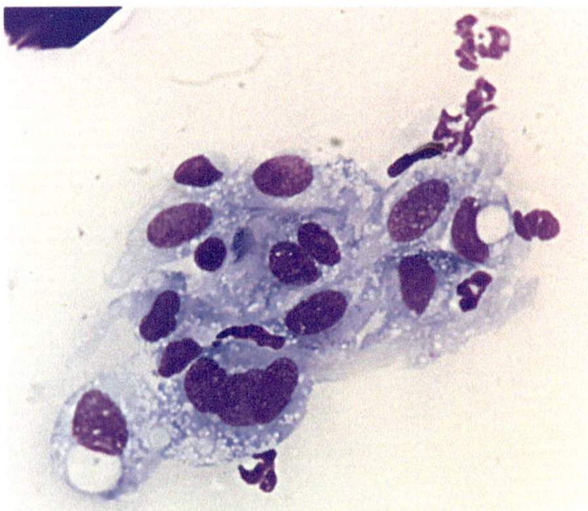

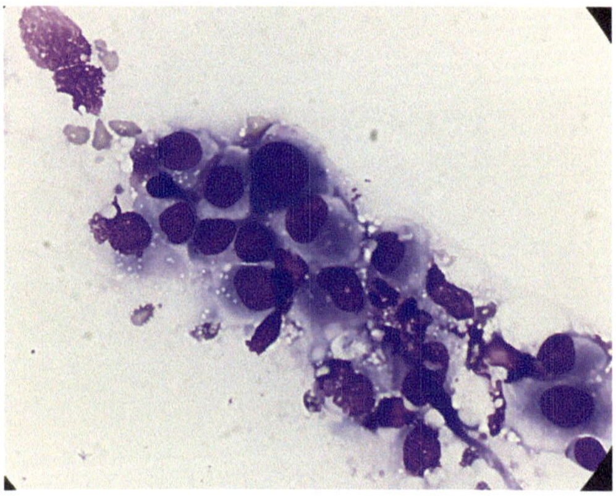

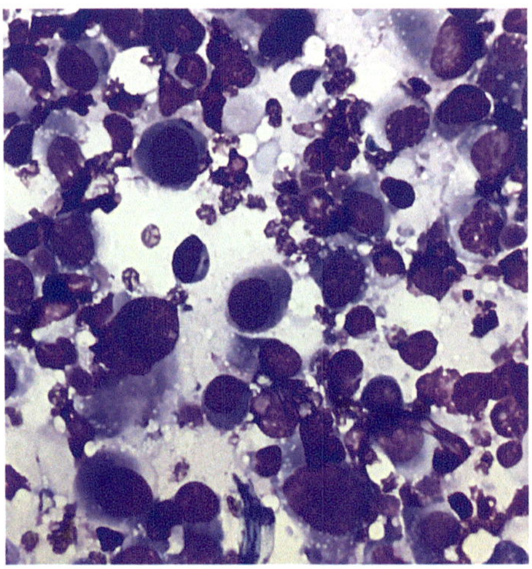

Figure 59.5. Images of fine-needle aspiration cytology of the nodules.

Answers Case 59

1 What type of skin pattern does this patient display, and what are the most likely diagnoses?

This patient has a nodular skin pattern. The differential diagnosis should include inflammatory or neoplastic nodules and nodular cystic lesions. Inflammatory nodules can be the result of bacterial infections (abscesses, atypical bacteria, botryomycosis), fungal infections (kerion, subcutaneous mycosis, systemic mycoses), parasitic infections (myiasis, leishmaniasis), and sterile inflammatory nodules (eosinophilic granuloma, foreign body granuloma, sterile nodular panniculitis, calcinosis circumscripta, sterile pyogranuloma, cutaneous histiocytosis, and nodular dermatofibrosis). In the case of neoplastic nodules the differential diagnosis is very broad (round, epithelial, and mesenchymal cell tumours). Cystic lesions can be follicular, sebaceous, or apocrine.

2 What cells are observed in the cytology and what type of pathology do they suggest?

Cytology shows a population of cells consisting of neutrophils and numerous large, round cells with clear, vacuolated cytoplasm and a round or oval nucleus with a histiocytic appearance.

The most probable diagnosis, based on the clinical signs and cytological findings, is cutaneous histiocytosis. Diagnosis was confirmed by dermatohistopathology.

Observations

Cutaneous histiocytosis is a rare, proliferative disorder that exclusively affects the skin. It is thought to be the result of a reactive, non-neoplastic process. It can affect dogs of 2 to 13 years of age. The clinical signs consist of multiple, erythematous cutaneous plaques or nodules (which in rare cases are subcutaneous), which can be alopecic and ulcerated. The nodules and plaques range in diameter from 1 to 5 cm, and are located on the head, neck, perineum, scrotum, and limbs (Fig. 59.6). They can spontaneously increase or decrease in size and appear in new areas.

Treatment is based on the administration of immunomodulatory drugs such as glucocorticoids, cyclosporine, the combination of doxycycline + nicotinamide, and leflunomide.

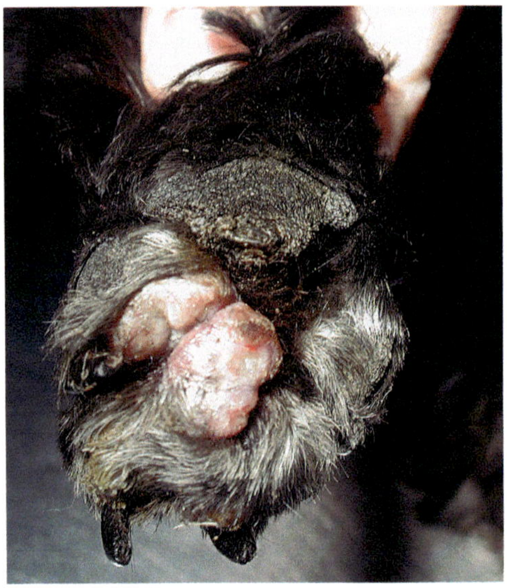

Figure 59.6. Interdigital nodules in a dog with cutaneous histiocytosis.

Case 60

Case presentation

A 2-year-old male English Bulldog was brought to the clinic with marked pruritus and lesions on the lateral aspect of the trunk (Fig. 60.1).

Questions

1 What are these lesions called and what is the underlying cause?

2 What differential diagnoses should be considered when this type of lesion appears?

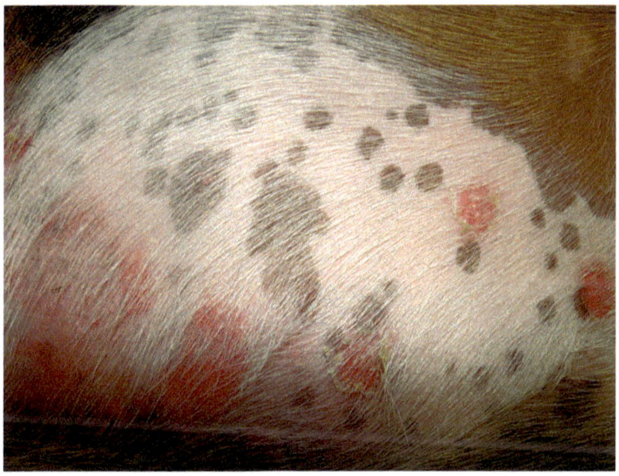

Figure 60.1. Pruritic lesions on the lateral aspect of the trunk.

Answers Case 60

1 What are these lesions called and what is the underlying cause?

These lesions are epidermal collarettes. This is a lesion typical of bacterial pyoderma. Disseminated superficial bacterial pyoderma or exfoliative superficial pyoderma is characterised by the presence of large collarettes, which may have a central erythematous or hyperpigmented area or an erythematous and crusted border (Figs. 60.2 and 60.3). In long-haired breeds such as the Scottish Shepherd (Collie), they are usually located on the trunk and give rise to areas of secondary alopecia. These lesions appear to be associated with the production of exfoliative toxins derived from the bacteria *Staphylococcus pseudintermedius*, resulting in loss of cohesion of the epidermal keratinocytes.

2 What differential diagnoses should be considered when this type of lesion appears?

Epidermal collarettes can appear, albeit infrequently, in pemphigus foliaceus, erythema multiforme, sterile eosinophilic pustulosis, pustular dermatophytosis, and demodicosis.

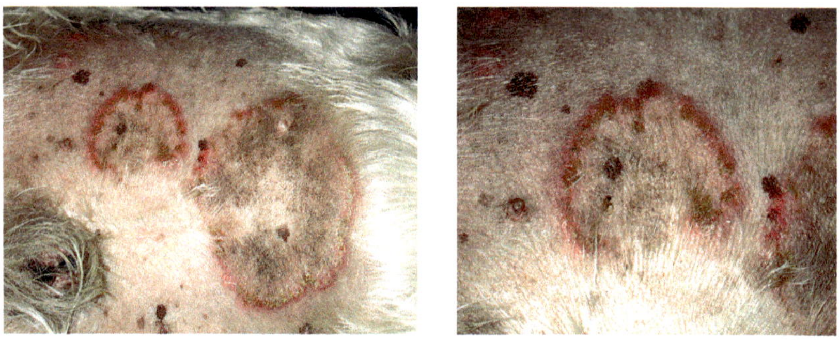

Figures 60.2 and 60.3. Large epidermal collarette on the skin of the abdomen of a dog with exfoliative superficial pyoderma.

Case 61

Case presentation

The owners of a castrated male French Bulldog, aged 11 years, brought him to the emergency room because he appeared depressed, with hyporexia that had appeared about 20 days earlier and breathing that was more forced and rapid than usual. The dog had no history of respiratory or cardiac disease, and his clinical history revealed only a chronic allergic condition and an osteoarthritic process affecting the lumbar vertebrae that had been treated with oral prednisone. Two weeks after the onset of the respiratory signs, a rapidly growing mass had appeared on the skin.

An increase in alveolar breath sounds was detected during the examination. A firm, violaceous cutaneous mass was observed on the lateral aspect of the neck (Figs. 61.1 and 61.2).

Thoracic radiography revealed a generalised interstitial-alveolar pattern (Figs. 61.3 and 61.4). Fine-needle aspiration cytology of the cutaneous mass was also performed (Figs. 61.5 and 61.6).

Questions

1. Taking into account the cytological findings, what is the most likely diagnosis of the cutaneous mass?
2. Could it be related to the dog's general condition?

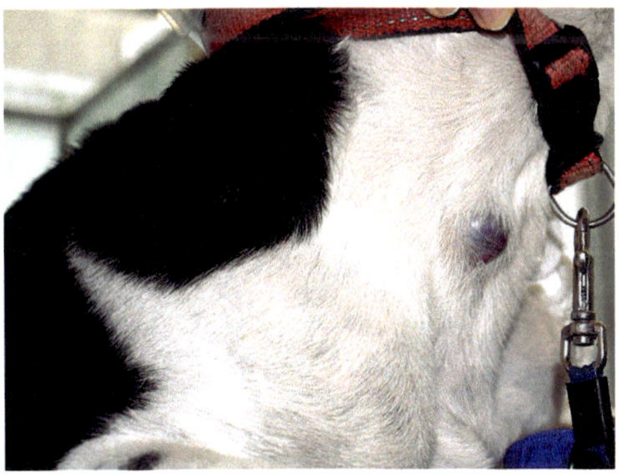
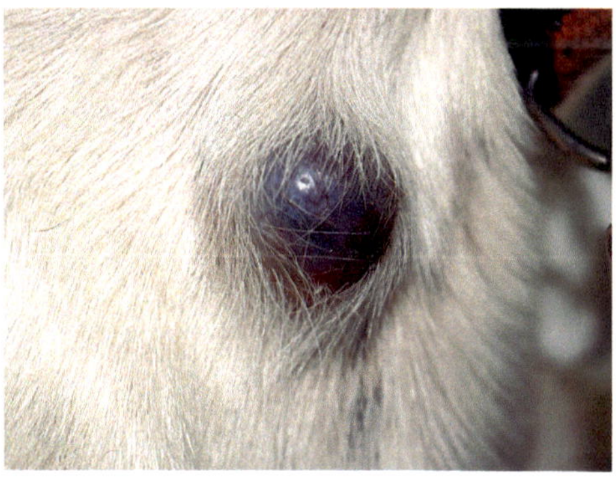

Figures 61.1 and 61.2. Violaceous cutaneous mass on the lateral aspect of the neck.

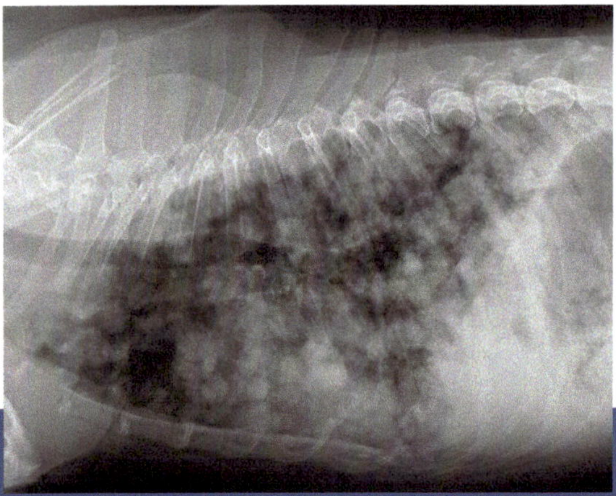
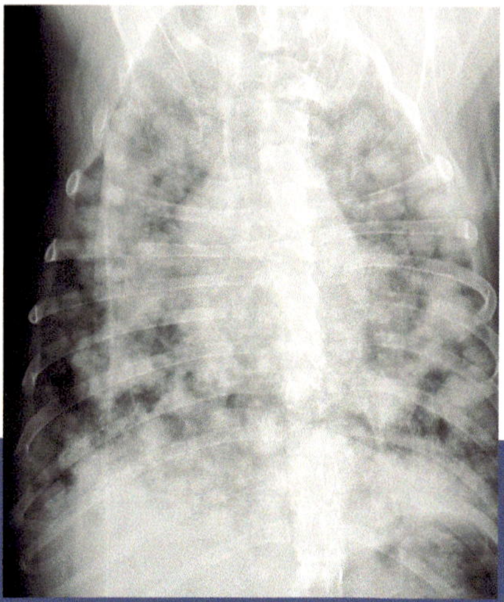

Figures 61.3 and 61.4. Lateral and ventrodorsal thoracic radiographs showing a generalised interstitial-alveolar pulmonary pattern.

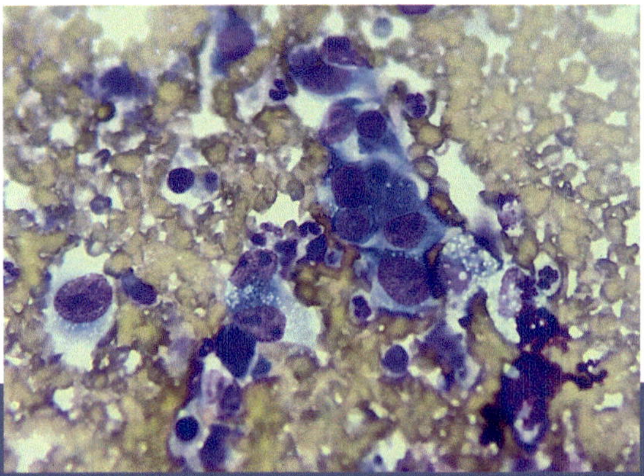
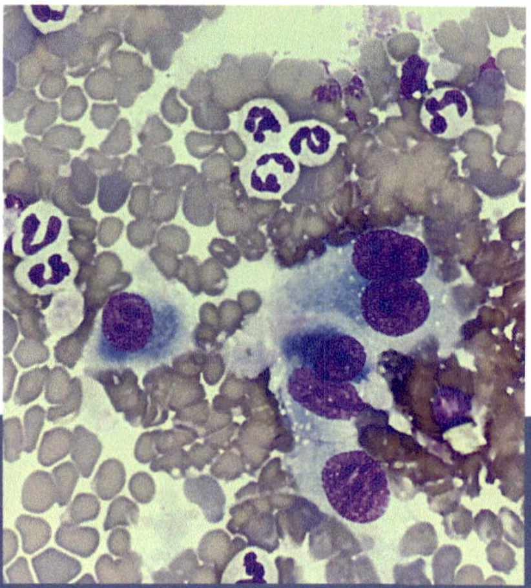

Figures 61.5 and 61.6. Images of fine-needle aspiration cytology of the cutaneous mass.

Answers Case 61

1 Taking into account the cytological findings, what is the most likely diagnosis of the cutaneous mass?

The cytology reveals the presence of moderate numbers of large tissue cells, with basophilic cytoplasm, poorly defined margins, and small vacuolisations. The cells exhibit characteristics compatible with malignancy such as anisokaryosis, multiple nuclei, and evident nucleoli (Fig. 61.7). The cytological and clinical characteristics of the mass are compatible with haemangiosarcoma.

2 Could it be related to the dog's general condition?

The respiratory distress and the radiographic findings are indicative of a neoplastic pulmonary process. The appearance of clinical signs in this case suggests that the cutaneous tumour and the pulmonary neoplasm may be related.

Given the poor prognosis, the owners refused further diagnostic tests and decided to euthanise the animal.

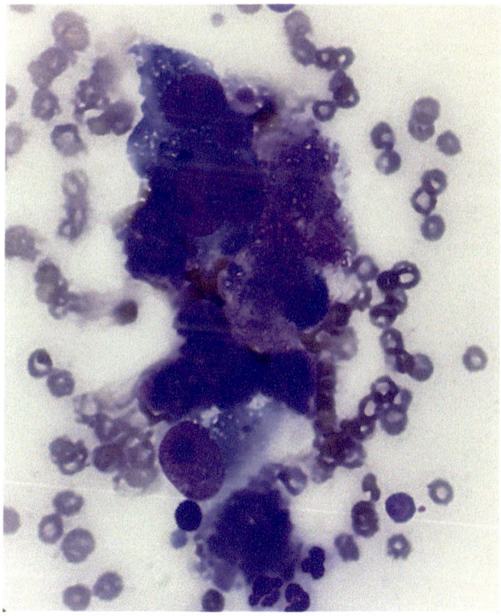

Figure 61.7. Cytological image of a cutaneous haemangiosarcoma showing marked signs compatible with malignancy, including anisokaryosis, multinucleated cells, and evident nucleoli.

Observations

Haemangiosarcoma (HSA) is a highly aggressive malignant tumour frequently observed in dogs. Primary HSA more often affects the spleen, the right atrium of the heart, the skin and subcutaneous tissue, and the liver, although primary forms have been described in the kidney, retroperitoneal space, muscle, bone, nasal and oral cavities, urinary bladder, and lungs.

Two forms are described for canine cutaneous HSA: cutaneous HSA caused by solar radiation, usually characterised by multiple lesions and affecting areas that dogs expose to the sun such as the skin of the abdomen (Fig. 61.8); and the cutaneous form unrelated to sun exposure, generally characterised by solitary cutaneous or subcutaneous masses.

The biological behaviour depends on the location of the primary tumour; tumours affecting the skin and subcutaneous tissue have a better prognosis than those in other locations. Metastasis can occur anywhere; liver, omentum, lungs, and skin. In this case, it is difficult to determine which is the primary tumour. However, the initial appearance of respiratory distress suggests that the skin tumour is secondary, caused by metastasis of a pulmonary neoplasm.

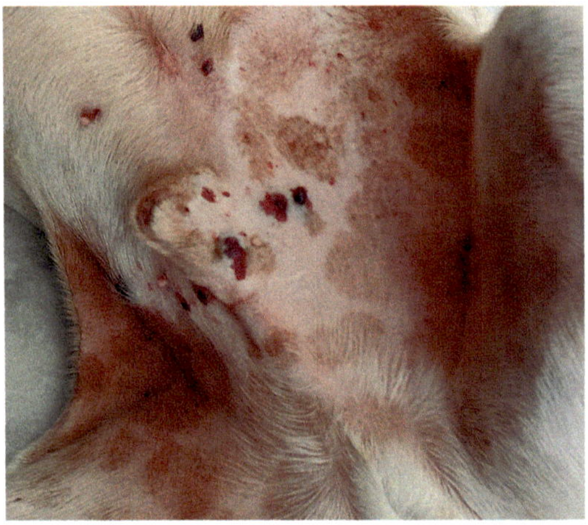

Figure 61.8. Cutaneous haemangiosarcomas on a dog's abdomen caused by sun exposure.

Case 62

Case presentation

The patient was a 7-year-old intact male Shih Tzu with inflammation of the skin of the digits of the left forepaw that had begun 4 months earlier. He had undergone an ultrasound to rule out foreign bodies and had been treated with an ointment containing corticosteroids and antibiotics, but showed no signs of improvement. He lived in a city apartment with no other animals. His owners had no skin lesions. He was fed a high-grade diet, and he had not been treated with external antiparasitic products.

The general examination revealed no findings of note, except for swelling of the second digit of the left forepaw. Examination of the skin revealed hyperpigmentation, lichenification on all digits of the left forepaw, and fistulous tracts with haemorrhagic exudate on the second digit (Fig. 62.1). The animal showed pain upon examination of the limb. The dermatological examination revealed no other findings of note.

Questions

1. What pathologies should be included in the differential diagnosis of this patient?
2. What diagnostic tests should be performed?

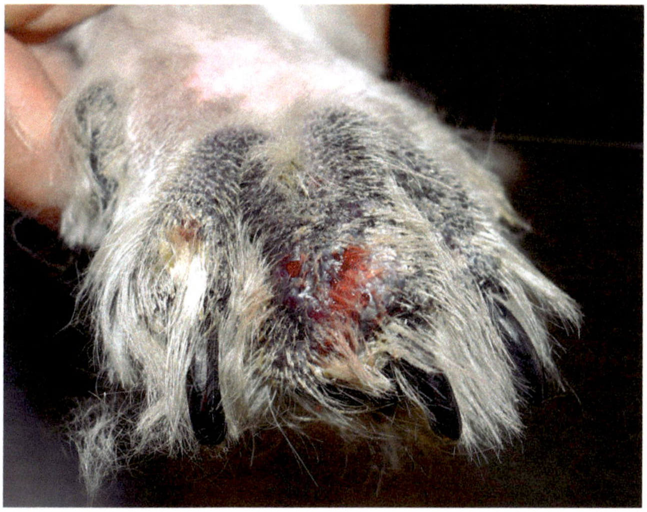

Figure 62.1. Appearance of the digits of the left forepaw after clipping. Lichenification, hyperpigmentation, and fistulas with haemorrhagic exudate are observed.

Answers Case 62

1 What pathologies should be included in the differential diagnosis of this patient?

The dog presents with inflammation of a digit with lichenification, hyperpigmentation, fistulous tracts with haemorrhagic exudate, and pain. All these clinical signs denote an inflammatory process affecting the deep layers of the skin and subcutaneous tissue. The differential diagnosis includes pododermatitis due to a deep pyoderma with or without demodicosis, deep mycosis, environmental trauma, foreign bodies, and neoplasm.

2 What diagnostic tests should be performed?

In this case, radiography of the digits showed soft tissue inflammation in the second digit. Cytology revealed the presence of neutrophils with intra- and extracellular bacteria (cocci), corresponding to a suppurative exudate. In the trichogram, numerous adult *Demodex canis* mites were detected (Fig. 62.2), while *Staphylococcus pseudintermedius* sensitive to enhanced penicillin and beta-lactam antibiotics grew in the bacterial culture.

The patient was treated with monthly oral fluralaner at a dose of 25 mg/kg for 2 months and oral amoxicillin/clavulanic acid (20 mg/kg every 12 hours) for 3 weeks. After 2 months, the inflammation and skin lesions had resolved, the skin scraping was negative, and only a change in skin colour was observed (Fig. 62.3).

Pododemodicosis is considered a generalised canine demodicosis and is associated with folliculitis and bacterial furunculosis. In this clinical case the primary cause that triggered the inflammatory process is unknown, although prolonged treatment with topical glucocorticoids may cause immunosuppression, favouring this process.

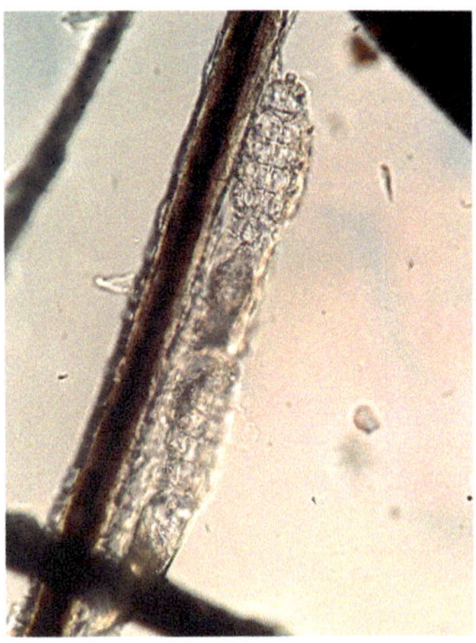

◀ Figure 62.2. Trichogram of the patient in which two adult *Demodex canis* mites are evident.

Figure 62.3. Appearance of the dog's limb 2 months after beginning treatment; the lesions have resolved. The change in hair colour may be due to the intense inflammatory process. ▶

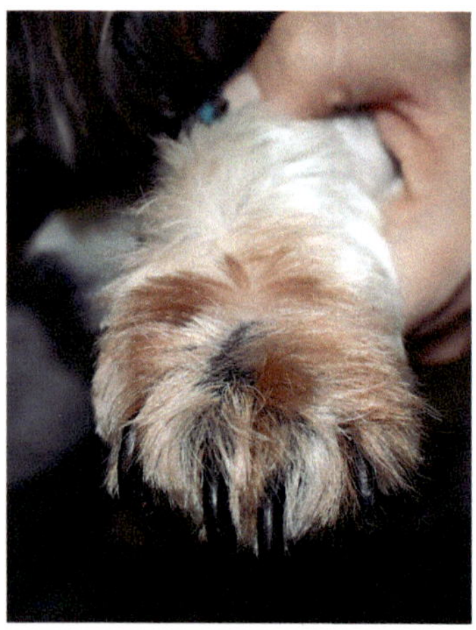

Case 63

Case presentation

An intact male French Bulldog of 2 years of age was brought to a dermatology clinic in the spring with signs of pruritus. The previous year, also in spring time, he had developed a pruritic condition that had persisted until the end of summer. His owners reported that he scratched his face and ears and continuously licked his legs. They had also observed lesions in the axillae and groin. No problems had been observed over the winter. The previous year his pruritus had been controlled with prednisone, but this medication caused vomiting and diarrhoea. The dog lived in a city apartment and his owners administered treatment to control for fleas and other external parasites throughout the year.

The dog presented with erythema on the muzzle and pinnae, and in the interdigital space. The eyelids were inflamed and alopecic, and excessive lacrimation was evident. Erythema, papules, and excoriation were observed on the axillae (Figs. 63.1–63.3).

Impression cytology of the affected skin was performed (Fig. 63.4).

Questions

1. How should the skin cytology be interpreted?
2. What can cause these recurrent skin lesions?
3. What treatments would be recommended?

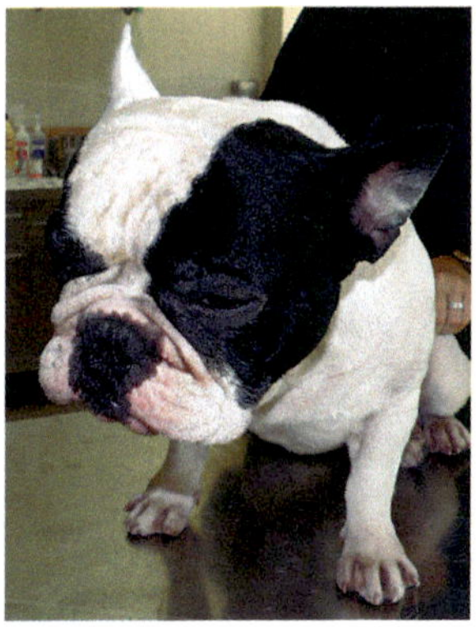

◀ Figure 63.1. Erythema affecting the muzzle, pinnae, and interdigital space. Lacrimation, blepharospasm, and alopecia of the eyelids.

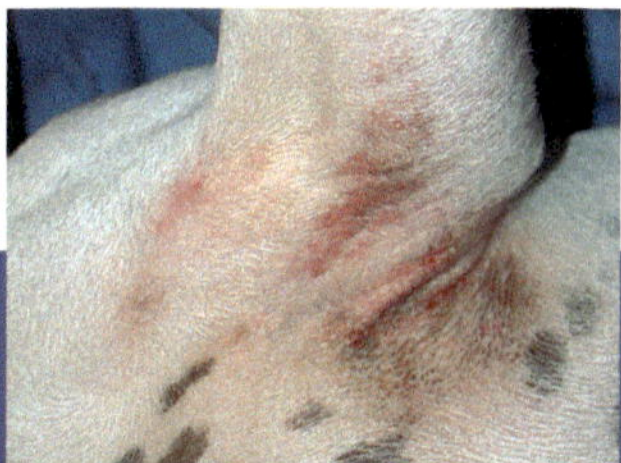

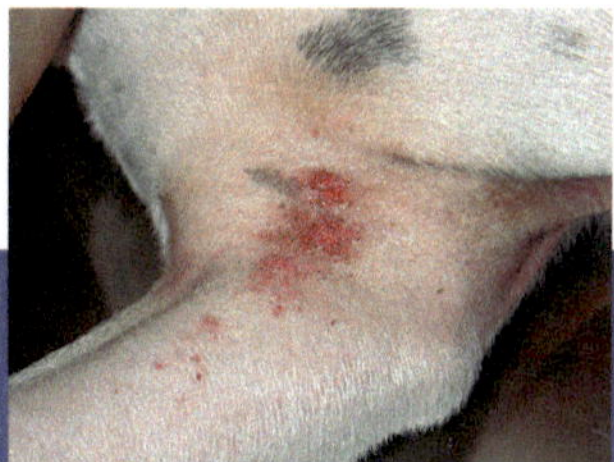

Figures 63.2 and 63.3. Erythema, papules, and excoriation on the axillae.

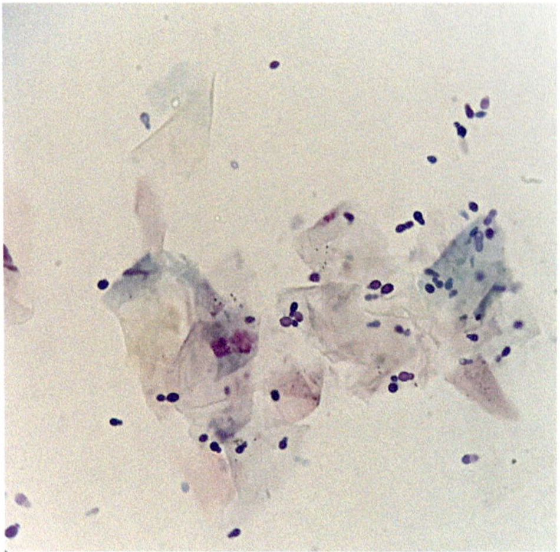

Figure 63.4. Impression cytology of the skin of the axillae.

Answers Case 63

1 How should the skin cytology be interpreted?

Skin cytology shows corneocytes and *Malassezia* spp., indicating *Malassezia* overgrowth.

2 What can cause these recurrent skin lesions?

The lesions could be caused by seasonal atopic dermatitis, since most of the clinical criteria are fulfilled in this case: appearance of clinical signs before 3 years of age; a dog that lives outdoors; pruritus that responds to corticosteroids; involvement of the pinnae with no lesions on the ear margin; and the absence of lesions in the thoracolumbar area. Other differential diagnoses of seasonal pruritus include flea-bite allergic dermatitis and allergic reactions to other parasites. The fact that this patient received antiparasitic treatment throughout the year increases the likelihood that this is a case of seasonal atopic dermatitis.

3 What treatments would be recommended?

For the treatment of seasonal atopic dermatitis it is recommended to use medications for the control of pruritus (e.g. oral oclacitinib) and topical glucocorticoids (e.g. hydrocortisone aceponate) in specific body areas and in those with little hair, such as the axillae. Secondary infections, caused either by *Malassezia* or bacteria, can be controlled with baths and the application of chlorhexidine and ketoconazole in the form of shampoos, lotions, or gels.

Case 64

Case presentation

A 1.5-year-old, castrated Labrador Retriever was brought to the veterinary surgeon with lesions on the muzzle. The lesions had appeared at 3 months of age and had very gradually worsened. The owners noticed some scaling, but had not noticed any wounds, and reported that the dog appeared unperturbed by the lesions. The dog lived in an apartment with a garden and was fed a high-grade diet. Neither his owners, nor the turtle with which he lived in the same apartment, had any skin lesions.

The results of the general examination were normal, and hyperkeratosis and small fissures were observed on the muzzle (Figs. 64.1 and 64.2). The appearance of the footpads and the rest of the skin was normal.

Impression cytology of the muzzle showed corneocytes, neutrophils, and intracellular and extracellular bacteria (cocci).

Questions

1 What is the most likely diagnosis of the lesions on the patient's nose?

2 How could the condition of the lesions be improved?

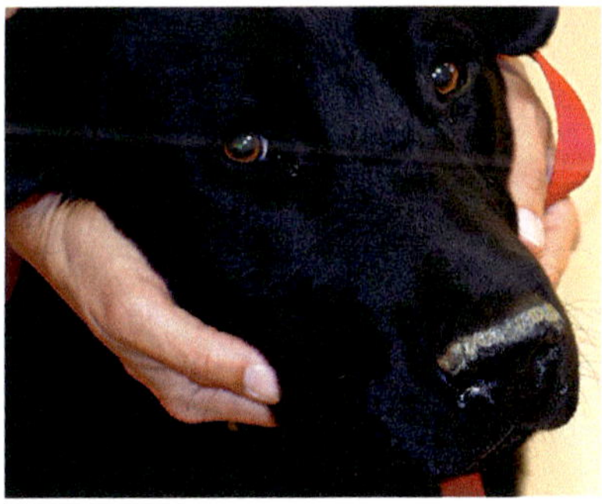

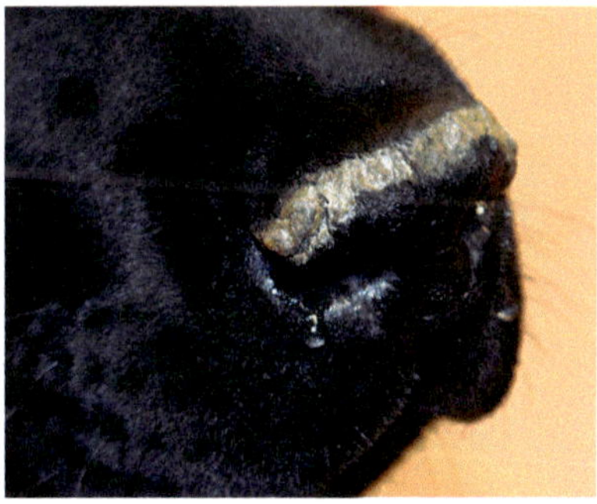

Figures 64.1 and 64.2. Hyperkeratosis on the muzzle of the patient.

Answers Case 64

1 What is the most likely diagnosis of the lesions on the patient's nose?

Nasal hyperkeratosis of slow progression, as seen in this patient, is characteristic of zinc-sensitive dermatosis, nasal parakeratosis of Labrador Retrievers, ichthyosis, and leishmaniasis. A more rapid progression is associated with pemphigus foliaceus/erythematosus, lupus erythematosus, drug reactions, and hepatocutaneous syndrome.

In this case, the most probable diagnosis is nasal parakeratosis of Labrador Retrievers, since the skin lesions exclusively affect the muzzle. This is an autosomal recessive hereditary disease of the Labrador Retriever breed and its crosses. The lesions appear between 3 months and 1 year of age and begin with a dry and rough proliferation of keratin on the nasal plane. Parakeratotic hyperkeratosis is observed in the histological examination. Lesions may develop on the footpads in older dogs (Fig. 64.3).

2 How could the condition of the lesions be improved?

Hyperkeratosis favours the appearance of fissures that become infected secondarily. This dog was treated with an antibiotic ointment and emollients and moisturisers, which improved the appearance of the muzzle (Fig. 64.4).

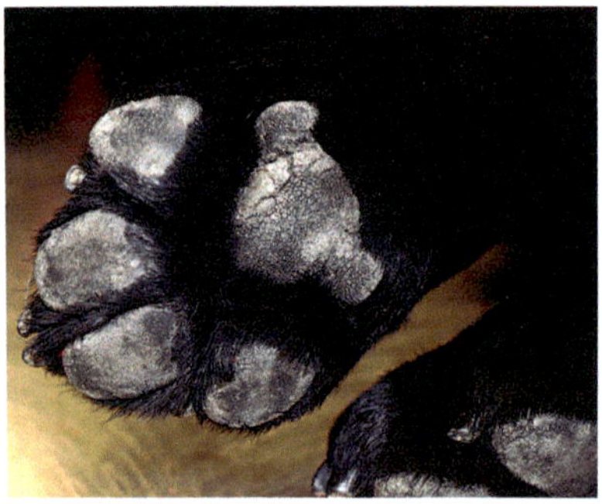

Figure 64.3. Hyperkeratosis on the footpads of a Labrador Retriever.

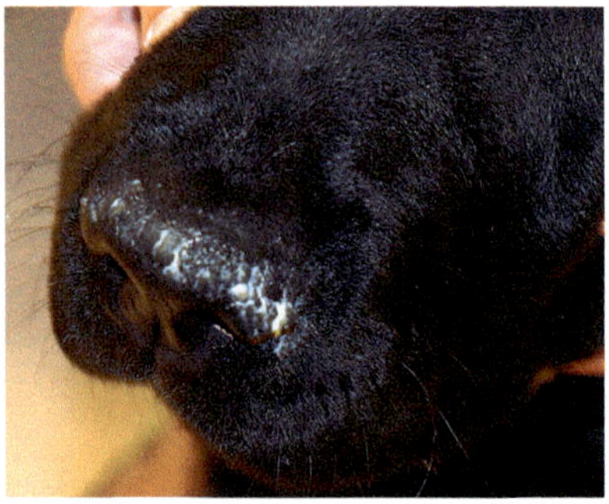

Figure 64.4. Appearance of the patient's muzzle 1 month after starting treatment with topical antibiotics and emollient and moisturising agents, including topical urea.

Case 65

Case presentation

A spayed Chihuahua bitch, aged 9 years, was brought to the clinic by her owner, who reported that the dog appeared to have lost hair. The owner reported that the dog's general condition was good, and that she appeared unperturbed by the loss of hair. The dog had been adopted 2 months earlier.

The results of the general examination were normal. In the dermatological examination, hypotrichosis and alopecia were observed in the preauricular area, the caudomedial area of the thighs, and on the ventral aspect of the neck and the ventral aspect of the trunk (Fig. 65.1). No other skin lesions were observed.

No infectious or parasitic agents were detected in the trichogram.

Questions

1 Is the alopecia presented by the patient inflammatory or noninflammatory?

2 What is the most likely cause of the alopecia?

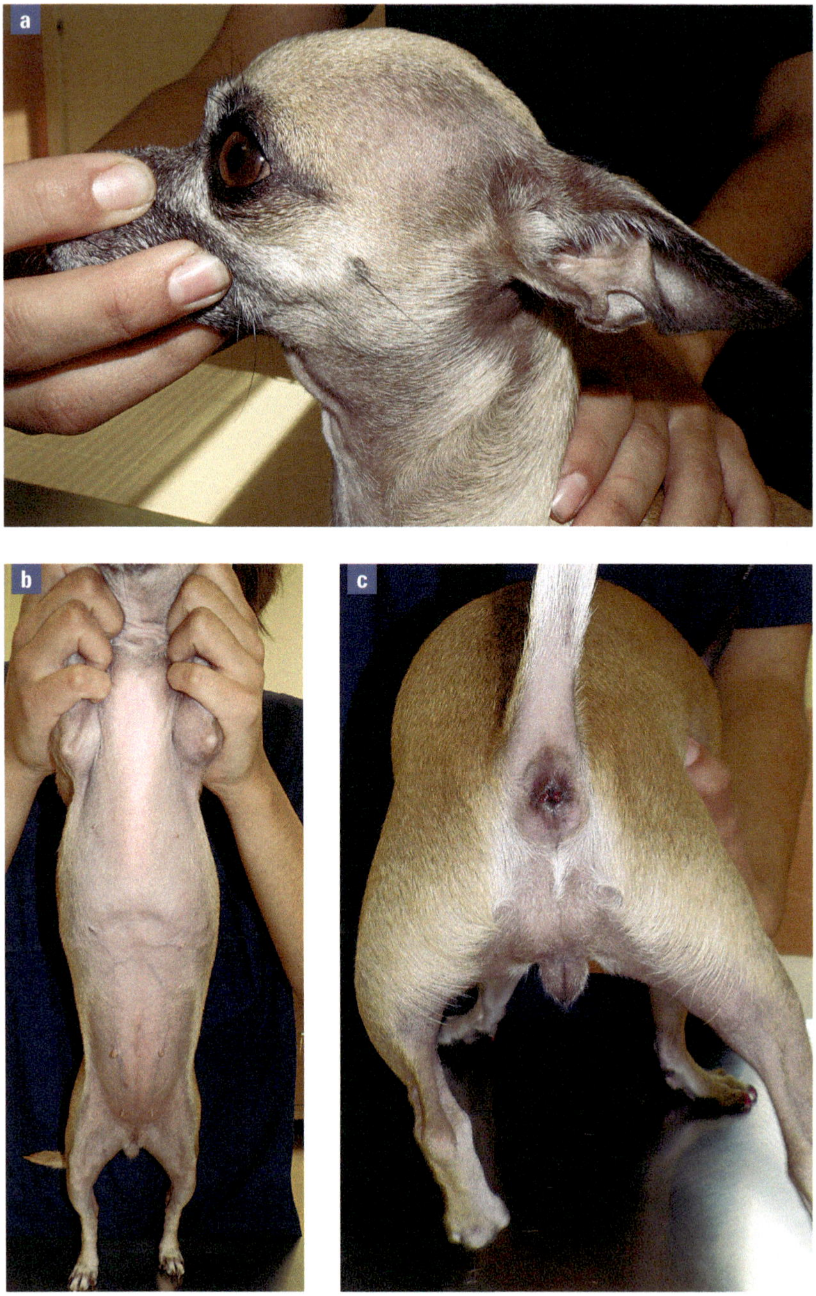

Figure 65.1. Hypotrichosis and alopecia in the preauricular area (a), on the ventral aspects of the neck and trunk (b), and in the caudomedial area of the thighs (c).

Answers Case 65

1 Is the alopecia presented by the patient inflammatory or noninflammatory?

The hair loss is noninflammatory, since no lesions indicative of inflammation (e.g. erythema, papules, pustules, crusts) are clinically evident.

2 What is the most likely cause of the alopecia?

Based on the clinical appearance, lesion distribution, and breed of the animal, this is likely a case of pattern alopecia. This is a disorder characterised by miniaturisation of the follicles and the diaphysis of the hair, without involvement of the adnexa. The hair is thinner and shorter than normal, and the size of the follicular bulb is reduced. It is a hereditary disorder in which animals are born with a normal coat of hair, but progressively develop hypotrichosis and alopecia with age.

There are several clinical syndromes:

- The first is alopecia of the pinnae, observed in Dachshunds (Fig. 65.2).
- The second is the form observed in the Portuguese Water Dog and the American Water Dog, with alopecia on the ventral aspect of the neck, caudomedial area of the thighs, and the tail.
- The third pattern alopecia syndrome is that which affects the caudal aspect of the thighs in Greyhounds (Fig. 65.3). It should be differentiated from Greyhound alopecia, in which hair loss affects the lateral aspect of the thighs and may have an endocrine basis.
- The fourth form, to which this clinical case corresponds, is the most common and is observed in the Chihuahua, Boston Terrier, Dachshund, Manchester Terrier, Whippet, and Greyhound. Beginning at 6 months of age dogs display symmetrical hair loss in the preauricular and postauricular areas, ventral aspect of the neck, ventral trunk area, and caudomedial aspect of the thighs (Fig. 65.4).

This is an aesthetic problem that has no effects on the animal's health. Some dogs respond to treatment with melatonin administered orally (3–9 mg/dog every 8 hours) or by subcutaneous implantation.

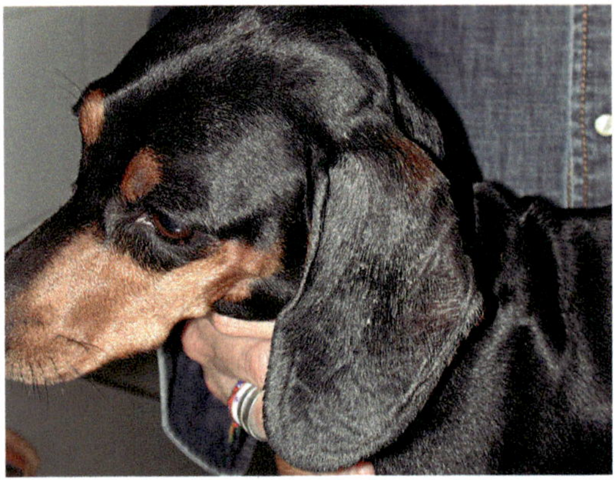

◄ Figure 65.2. Hypotrichosis and alopecia of the pinna of a Dachshund.

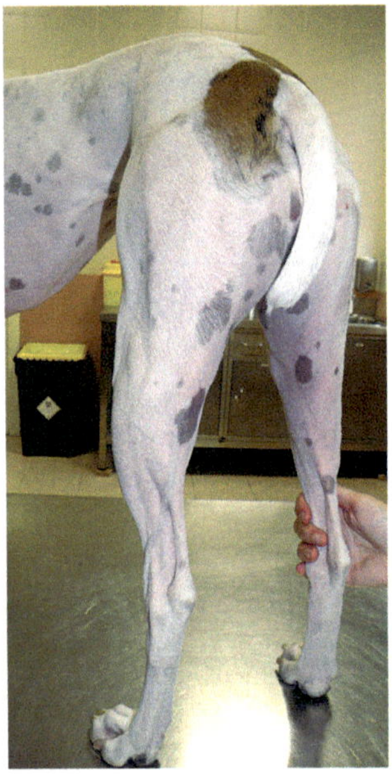

Figure 65.3. Greyhound with pattern alopecia affecting the caudal aspects of the thighs.

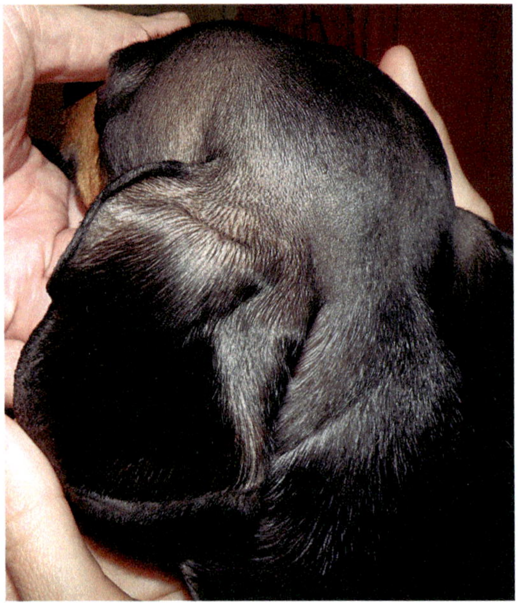

Figure 65.4. Preauricular and postauricular alopecia in a Dachshund with pattern alopecia.

Case 66

Case presentation

The patient was a spayed female domestic shorthair cat, aged 6 years, with suppurative patches on the skin of the inguinal area that had appeared 6 months earlier. The cat licked the lesions regularly. She had shown some improvement after administration of injectable corticosteroids, but 15 days after the injection the skin lesions had reappeared. She lived in an apartment with no other animals and no access to the outdoors. Her diet consisted of commercial cat food and she had not been treated with any external antiparasitic agents.

Examination revealed the presence of erythematous and highly exudative plaques on the skin of the abdomen, distributed linearly (Fig. 66.1).

Cytology of the lesions showed neutrophils with toxic changes, with the presence of intra- and extracellular bacteria (Fig. 66.2), as well as moderate numbers of eosinophils (Fig. 66.3).

Questions

1. What lesions are observed in this patient?
2. How can they be treated?

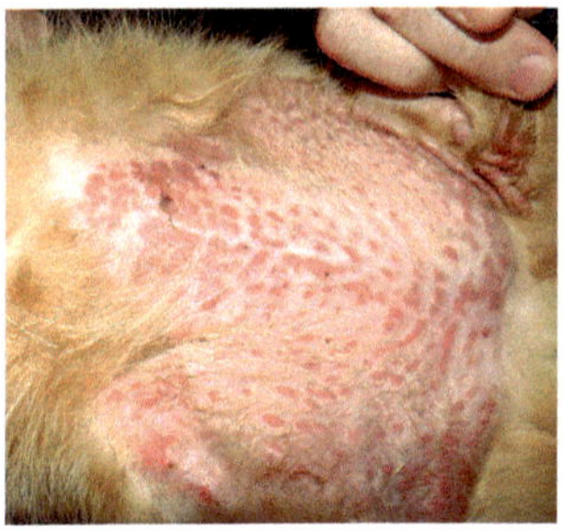

Figure 66.1. Erythematous and exudative plaques on the skin of the patient's abdomen.

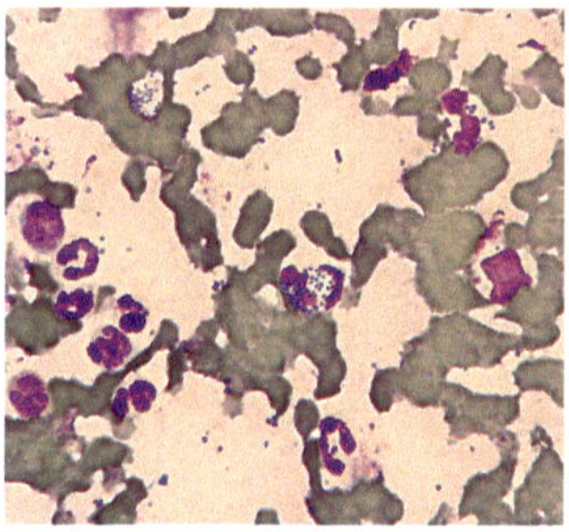

Figure 66.2. Cytology of purulent exudate containing intra- and extracellular bacteria (cocci).

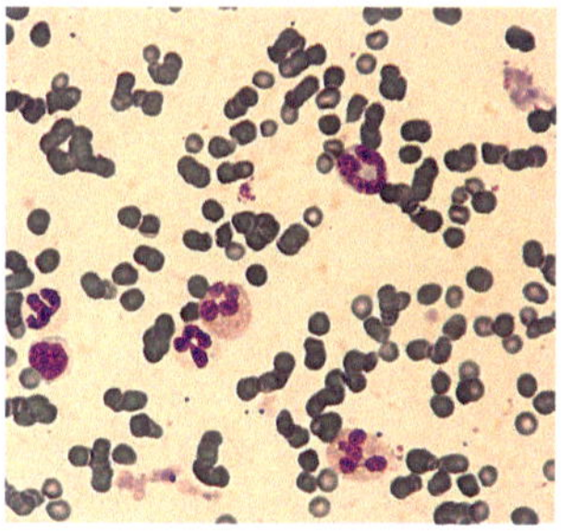

Figure 66.3. Cytological sample obtained from the lesion containing polymorphonuclear neutrophils and eosinophils.

Answers Case 66

1 What lesions are observed in this patient?

The lesions observed in this cat are eosinophilic plaques. This highly pruritic lesion is relatively common in cats; it is thought that both the pruritus itself and the consequent licking contribute to the development and persistence of the lesions. The plaques can be solitary or multiple, and are usually well defined, elevated, erythematous, highly exudative eroded or ulcerated lesions with foci of necrosis (Figs. 66.4 and 66.5). The distribution of the plaques is usually linear or oval with the longitudinal axis oriented in the direction in which the cat licks a given area of the body (Fig. 66.6). The majority are located on the skin of the abdomen and on the medial aspects of the thighs.

Cytology of the lesions shows eosinophils and neutrophils with intracellular bacteria. Secondary infections are very frequent and appear to play an important role in this pathology.

2 How can they be treated?

The recommended treatment is systemic antibiotic administration for 3 or 4 weeks and oral glucocorticoids in decreasing doses.

In cases of feline pruritus, it is recommended to carry out a complete and systematic diagnostic protocol to determine the origin.

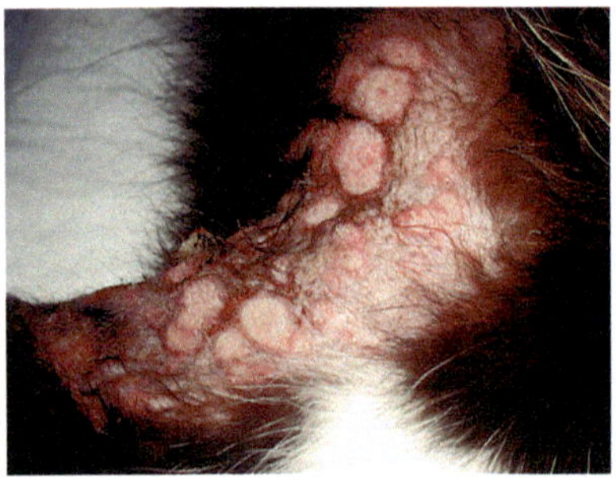
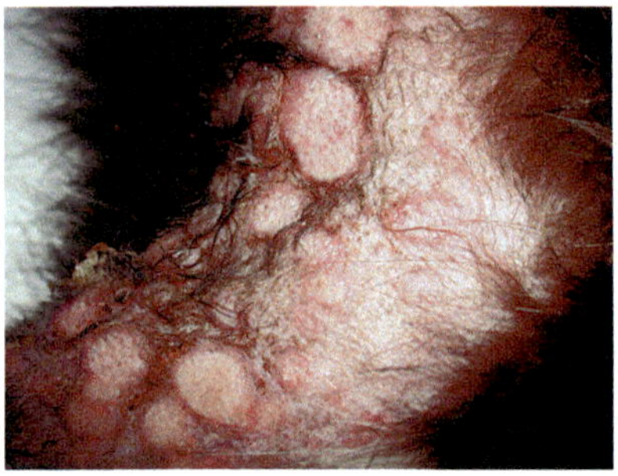

Figures 66.4 and 66.5. Elevated, well-defined, erythematous and eroded plaques on the medial aspect of a cat's thigh.

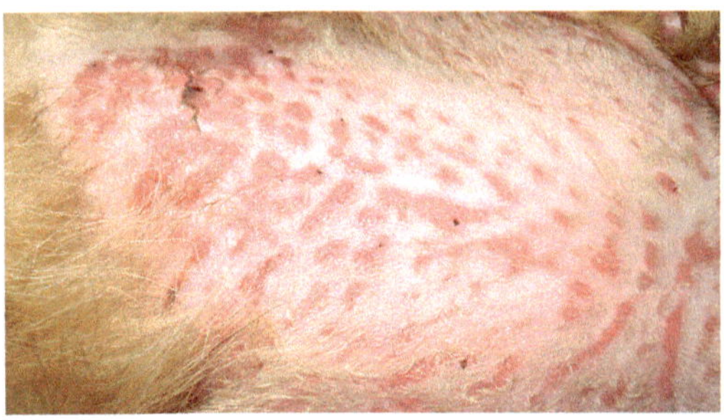

Figure 66.6. Distribution of the plaques in a linear or oval pattern.

Case 67

Case presentation

An intact mongrel bitch was brought to the emergency department with skin lesions of acute onset that progressively worsened, affecting the inner aspects of both forelimbs. The animal was prostrate and very weak. Fever (39.8 °C), tachypnoea, tachycardia, and pain in the limbs were observed in the examination.

The skin of the inner aspect of the forelimbs was clipped to better observe the extent of the lesions. This revealed erythema, exudation, erosion, and numerous areas of necrosis with macerated, devitalised, and greyish black skin (Figs. 67.1–67.3). These areas were surrounded by erythema and oedema and caused significant pain on palpation. The forelimbs were swollen and inflamed. Exudate cytology revealed the presence of neutrophils with large numbers of intra- and extracellular bacteria (cocci and bacilli).

Owing to the necrotic and devitalised appearance of the lesions and their widespread distribution, surgical debridement with sampling for culture and antibiogram were recommended. The surgical examination revealed the presence of macerated subcutaneous tissue that was easily separated from the fascia.

Questions

1 What is the most likely diagnosis, taking into account the clinical signs and surgical findings?

2 What organisms have been associated with this pathology?

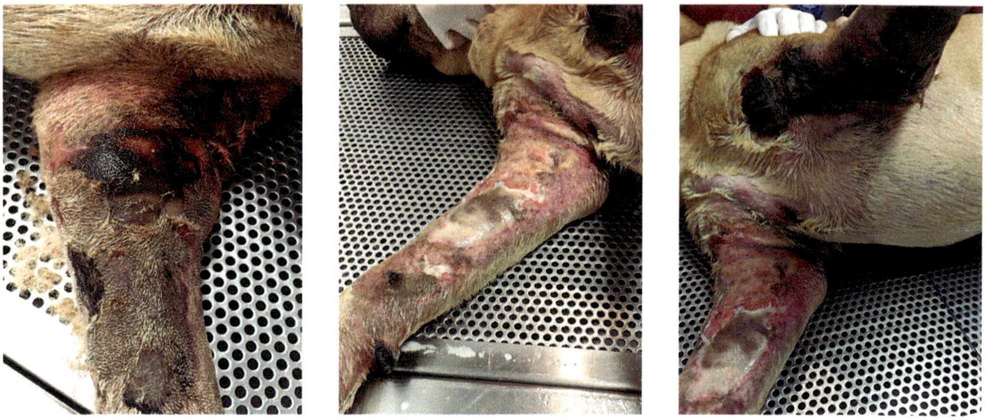

Figures 67.1–67.3. Erythema and oedema with patches of greyish-black skin on the inner aspects of both limbs of the patient.

Answers Case 67

1 What is the most likely diagnosis, taking into account the clinical signs and surgical findings?

The clinical picture and surgical findings are compatible with cellulitis with necrotising fasciitis.

Necrotising fasciitis is a rare infection of rapidly progressive course that affects the skin, the subcutaneous tissue, the superficial fascia, and occasionally the deep fascia. Thrombosis in the subcutaneous microcirculation gives rise to tissue necrosis, systemic toxicity, and a high mortality rate.

2 What organisms have been associated with this pathology?

In veterinary medicine this pathology has been associated with *Streptococcus canis* infection, although a synergistic action between aerobic and anaerobic bacteria appears to be involved. While it is commonly associated with trauma, it can also occur in the absence of trauma. Aggressive and early treatment with surgical debridement and systemic antibiotic therapy can save the patient's life. Treatment with antibiotics with activity against anaerobic bacteria (e.g. clindamycin or metronidazole) is recommended.

Case 68

Case presentation

A 10-year-old spayed Golden Retriever bitch was brought to the clinic by her owners, who reported that the animal trembled and was more tired than usual. In the dermatological examination, alopecia with hyperpigmentation was observed on the nasal bridge (Fig. 68.1). The patient appeared unperturbed by the alopecia.

Questions

1. What pathologies can cause noninflammatory alopecia in this location?
2. What tests can be performed to confirm the diagnosis?

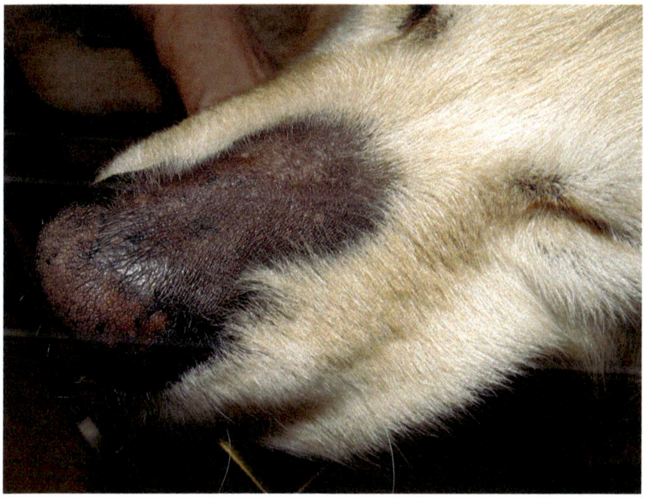

Figure 68.1. Alopecia and hyperpigmentation on the nasal bridge of the patient.

Answers Case 68

1 What pathologies can cause noninflammatory alopecia in this location?

Hypothyroidism and cyclic flank alopecia can cause noninflammatory alopecia of the nasal bridge. In this case, alopecia is associated with systemic clinical signs, suggesting hypothyroidism.

In the early stages of hypothyroidism, alopecia can be focal, multifocal, symmetrical, or asymmetrical. Hypotrichosis or alopecia affect areas of friction, such as pressure points on the ventral aspect of the abdomen, the perineum, and the tail. Unlike other endocrinopathies, alopecia in hypothyroidism can affect the face, nasal bridge, and pinnae (Fig. 68.2). In large and giant breeds, alopecia may appear on the lateral aspects of the extremities (Fig. 68.3). As the disease becomes chronic, hair loss can spread, acquiring a more symmetrical pattern.

2 What tests can be performed to confirm the diagnosis?

Definitive diagnosis of hypothyroidism requires a thyroid biopsy, but this technique is rarely used. Clinically, hypothyroidism is diagnosed based on the medical history, clinical signs, and the results of blood tests, urinalysis, skin biopsy, and thyroid tests. The classic forms of hypothyroidism present with mild nonregenerative anaemia, hypercholesterolaemia and hypertriglyceridaemia, increases in serum creatine kinase (CK) levels, and slight increases in alkaline phosphatase (ALP), lactate dehydrogenase (LDH), and aspartate-aminotransferase (AST/GOT). The skin biopsy shows changes consistent with an endocrinopathy, such as orthokeratotic hyperkeratosis, keratosis and follicular atrophy, epidermal melanosis, hair follicle telogenisation, excessive trichilemmal keratinisation, and atrophy of the sebaceous glands. Other histological findings suggestive of hypothyroidism include vacuolation of the piloerector muscles, increased levels of dermal mucin, and epidermal hypertrophy.

In dogs, low serum levels of total T_4 and elevated TSH levels are compatible with hypothyroidism. If the results are not conclusive, it is necessary to resort to determination of free T_4 levels by equilibrium dialysis.

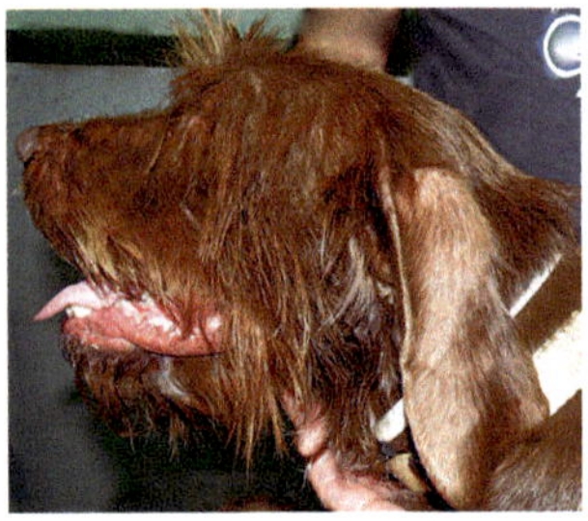

Figure 68.2. Alopecia on the pinna of a dog with hypothyroidism.

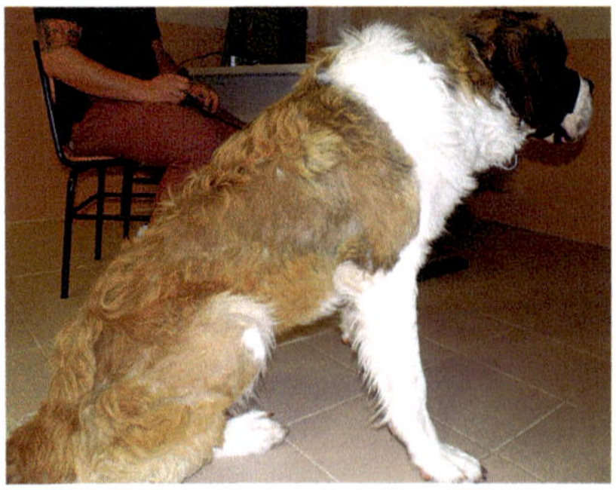

◀ Figure 68.3. Hypotrichosis on the lateral aspect of the thorax and external aspect of the thigh in a Saint Bernard with hypothyroidism.

Case 69

Case presentation

A 3-year-old intact male Labrador was brought to the clinic by his owner, who reported that he had developed orange crusts on the skin of his face. The dog had generalised pruritus. The owner was a forest ranger who lived in the Spanish province of Burgos.

Papular skin lesions on the abdomen, the eyelid, and the nasal bridge were observed in the examination (Fig. 69.1). Bright orange scaling on the skin of the eyelids was observed (Figs. 69.2 and 69.3). The parasite shown in Figures 69.4 and 69.5 was detected in the trichogram.

Questions

1. What parasite is this?
2. What is the treatment for this parasitosis?

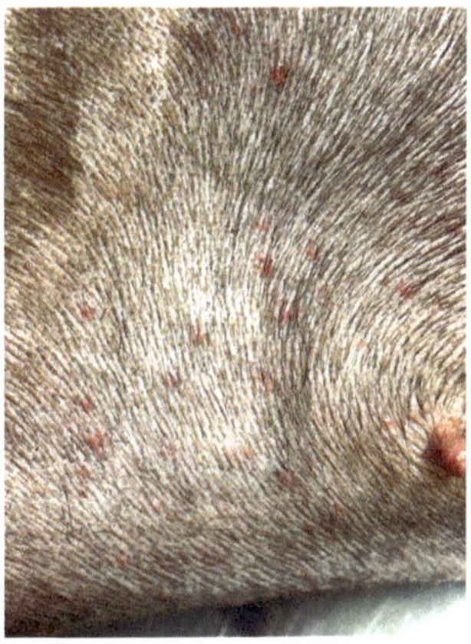

◄ Figure 69.1. Papules on the skin of the patient's abdomen.

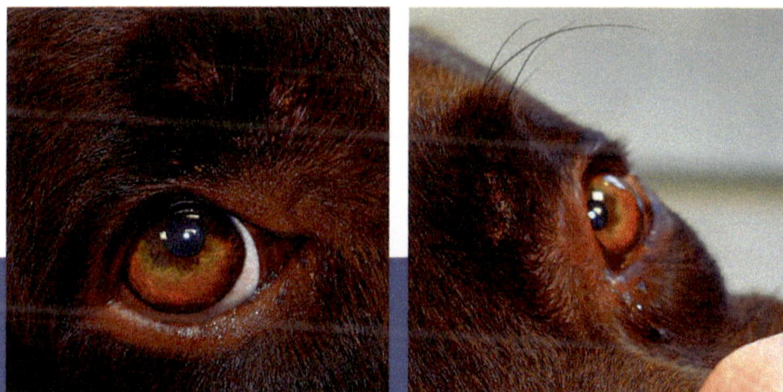

Figures 69.2 and 69.3. Bright orange spots on the eyelid.

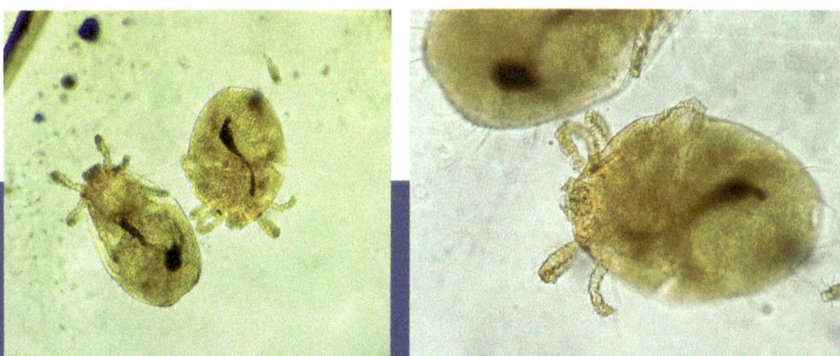

Figures 69.4 and 69.5. Mites observed in the trichogram.

Answers Case 69

1 What parasite is this?

This is *Neotrombicula autumnalis* or the harvest mite. This parasite is found worldwide in habitats ranging from semi-desert to marshland. It can live freely or parasitise plants or other arthropods. The larva feeds on vertebrate hosts, which are usually wild, although farm animals, pets, and people can become inadvertently infected. Eggs in the soil hatch and release larvae that climb vegetation to gain access to birds and mammals that pass by. Parasitisation is seasonal, between the end of summer and autumn, although it can last all year round in warm and temperate climates.

The larvae have an intense bright orange colour and an oval shape (Fig. 69.6). They are found mainly in areas of skin that make contact with the ground (digits, limbs, head, ears, and skin of the abdomen). The larvae can be observed as bright orange or yellow spots grouped in papules (Figs. 69.2 and 69.3). The degree of pruritus is variable and secondary lesions caused by scratching (e.g. excoriations, alopecia, scaling, and crusting) may appear.

2 What is the treatment for this parasitosis?

Affected patients should be treated with antiparasitics applied every 1 or 2 weeks either in spray form or via pipettes (spot-on). It has been reported that 0.25 % fipronil spray is effective for the treatment and prevention of trombiculiasis.

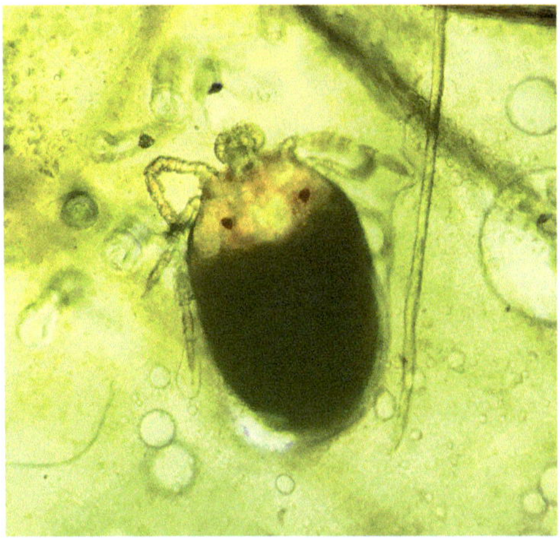

Figure 69.6. *Neotrombicula autumnalis* larva.

Case 70

Case presentation

A 1.5 year-old, intact male Yorkshire Terrier was referred to the reference veterinary hospital for imaging tests; his veterinary surgeon suspected a portosystemic shunt. At 7 months of age, the dog began biting his hindlimbs and tail. He bit and licked, but did not scratch the area in question, and the owners noticed only a decrease in the amount of hair in the area, but no other skin lesions. They were unsure whether this was due to hair falling out or being removed by the dog.

The animal had been purchased from a private individual, and had fleas and intestinal parasites that had been treated by the owners' usual veterinary surgeon. The dog had received medical treatment for a possible shunt, and showed no clinical signs of this pathology.

The results of the general examination were normal. The dog presented with hypotrichosis in the thoracolumbar area and on the lateral aspects of the thighs (Figs. 70.1 and 70.2). No other lesions were observed. No parasitic or infectious agents were detected following brushing and a trichogram.

Questions

1 How can we determine whether hypotrichosis is due to self-induced damage of the hair or caused by hair falling out?

2 What would be the most likely diagnoses in the event that the hair loss is self-induced?

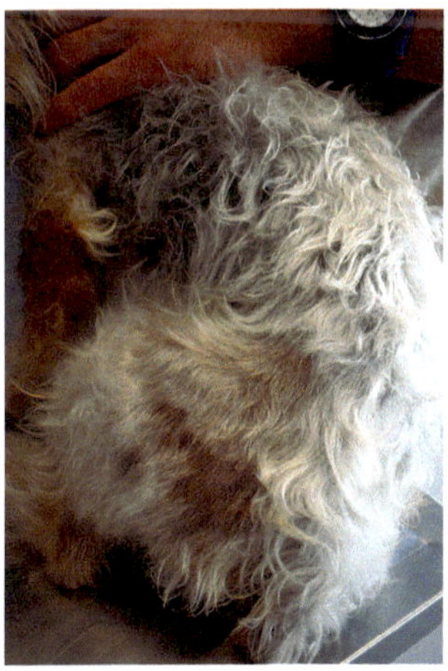

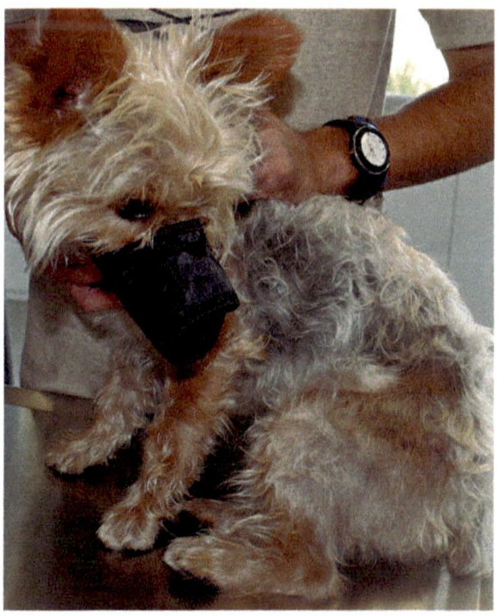

Figures 70.1 and 70.2. Hypotrichosis in the thoracolumbar area and on the lateral aspect of the patient's thigh.

Answers Case 70

1 How can we determine whether hypotrichosis is due to self-induced damage of the hair or caused by hair falling out?

In this case, the trichogram is a very useful diagnostic tool. Examination of the hair revealed nodular lesions in the hair shaft that could result in breakage (trichoclasia or trichorrhexis nodosa) (Fig. 70.3). The hair tips had a splayed appearance (trichoptilosis) (Figs. 70.4 and 70.5).

These alterations suggest that the hair loss is induced by trauma. Hypotrichosis can be self-induced or caused by aggressive environmental factors such as the use of antiparasitic products or aggressive cosmetics. In cases of self-induced hypotrichosis, the differential diagnosis should include pruritic conditions and behavioural disorders that cause compulsive licking, although sometimes these two pathologies can be associated.

2 What would be the most likely diagnoses in the event that the hair loss is self-induced?

The following are the most probable causes of pruritus, considering the animal's age and the distribution of the lesions: flea bite allergy; hypersensitivity to intestinal parasites; presence of other parasites such as *Cheyletiella*; and food intolerance or allergy. Pruritus due to liver disease, although common in humans, is very rare in canine species. In this patient, the pruritus disappeared following surgical resolution of the shunt, without the need for any other type of treatment.

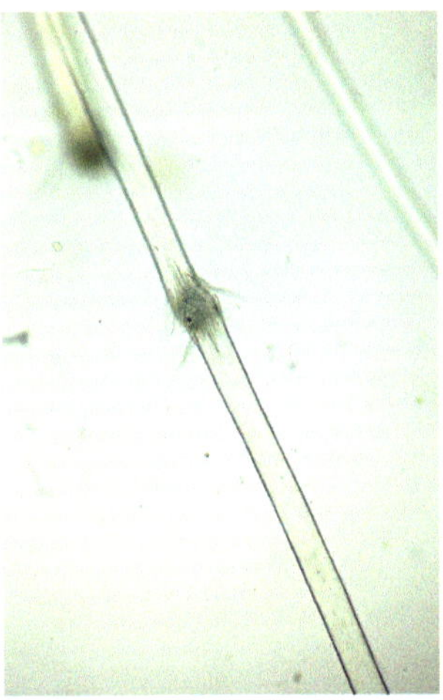

◄ Figure 70.3. Nodular lesion causing breakage of the hair shaft (trichoclasia or trichorrhexis nodosa).

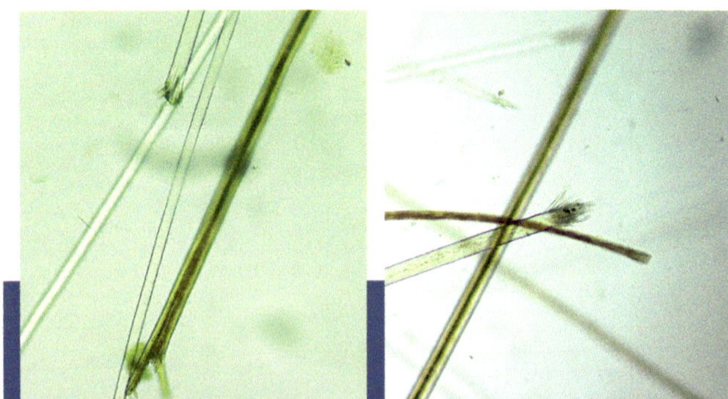

Figures 70.4 and 70.5. Frayed and broken hair tips (trichoptilosis).

Case 71

Case presentation

A 9-year-old male mongrel dog with small plaques on his face and body was referred by the hospital's oncology service. In addition, he had lost his whiskers (Figs. 71.1–71.3). The dog had begun chemotherapy with doxorubicin 6 months earlier, but appeared healthy, and had normal blood test results.

Questions

1 Could the hair loss be due to doxorubicin treatment?

2 What other dermatological disorders are associated with chemotherapy?

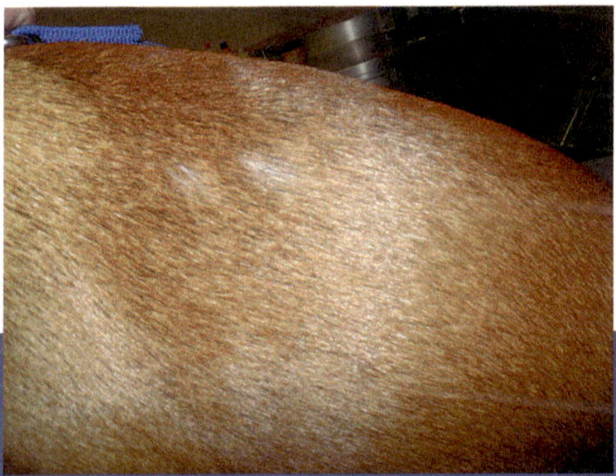

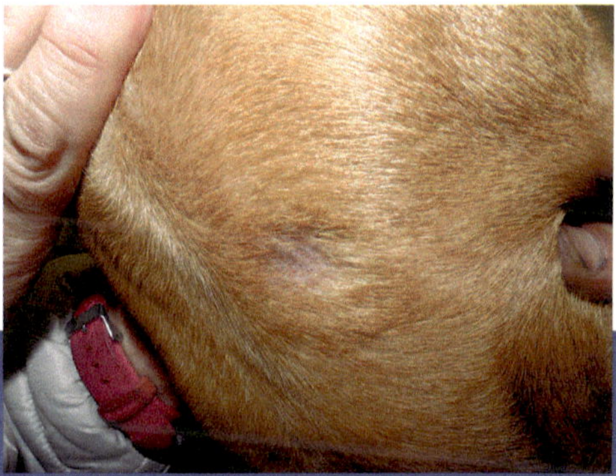

Figures 71.1 and 71.2. Multifocal alopecia on the trunk and face.

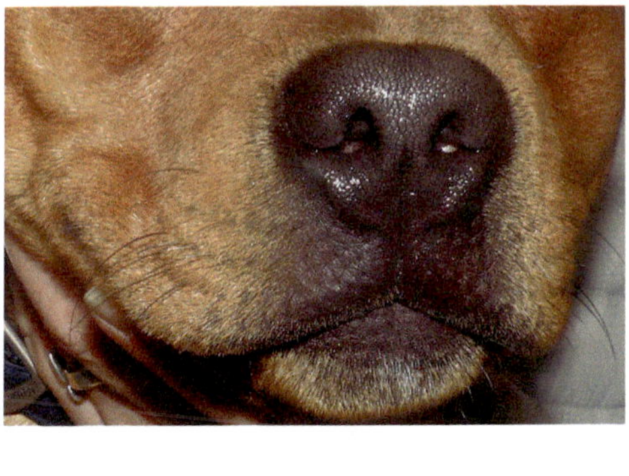

Figure 71.3. Absence of whiskers.

Answers Case 71

1 Could the hair loss be due to doxorubicin treatment?

Chemotherapy-induced alopecia is very common in human medicine and has been recently described in veterinary oncology. The underlying pathophysiological process is not completely known, and no effective treatment has been identified to date. Doxorubicin is known to induce apoptosis of the precursor cells of the hair bulb in anagen phase, resulting in abrupt narrowing of the hair follicle. This results in anagen effluvium, caused by breakage of the fragile hair once it reaches the surface of the skin (Fig. 71.4). It has been reported that almost 20 % of dogs treated with doxorubicin can develop alopecia.

2 What other dermatological disorders are associated with chemotherapy?

In addition to alopecia, oncological medications can cause maculopapular eruptions, erythroderma and exfoliative dermatitis, urticaria-like reactions, angioedema, and erythema multiforme. Pruritic conditions can also be induced by chemotherapeutic agents such as carboplatin, cyclophosphamide, methotrexate, vincristine, and toceranib. Opioid medications and associated analgesics such as morphine, tramadol, fentanyl, buprenorphine, and naltrexone are an important group of drugs that produce pruritus and are associated with oncological treatment.

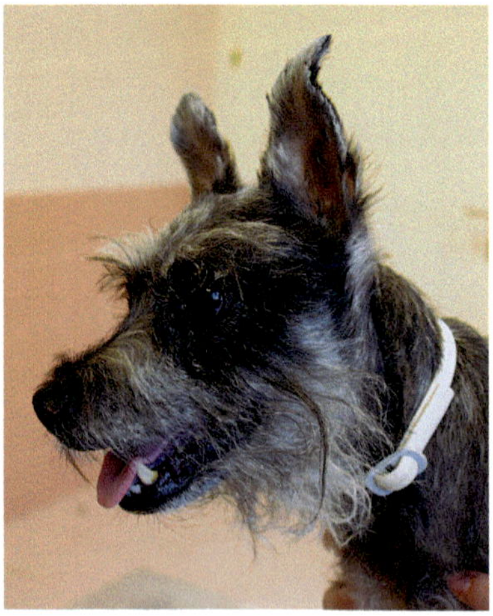

Figure 71.4. Hypotrichosis on the face of a Schnauzer treated with doxorubicin.

Case 72

Case presentation

A 7-year-old male domestic shorthair cat was brought to the clinic with mange that did not respond to acaricide treatment. Clinical signs had first appeared 4 months earlier and, despite treatment with selamectin, new lesions had appeared.

In the general examination the animal appeared depressed and had a fever. Examination of the skin revealed crusts on the pinnae, nasal bridge, muzzle, and around the nails (Figs. 72.1–72.3).

Questions

1. What pathologies should be included in the differential diagnosis of this case?
2. What diagnostic tests should be performed?

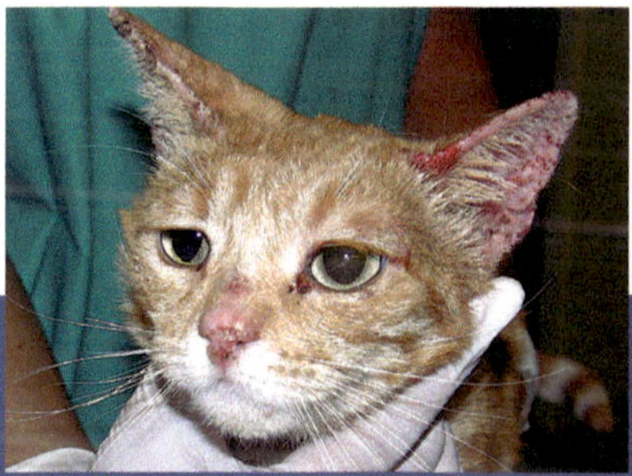

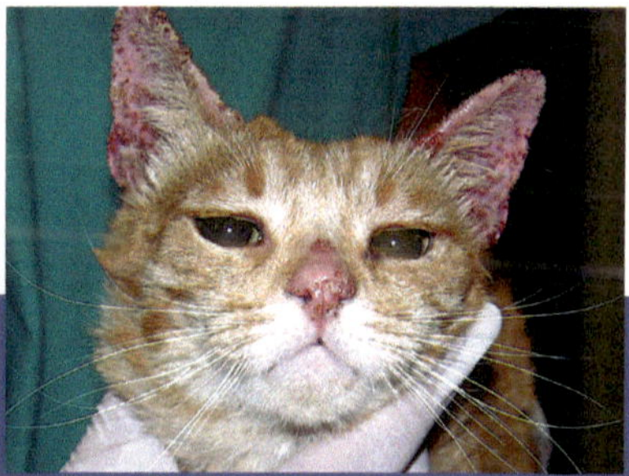

Figures 72.1 and 72.2. Crusted lesions on the pinnae, muzzle, and nasal bridge.

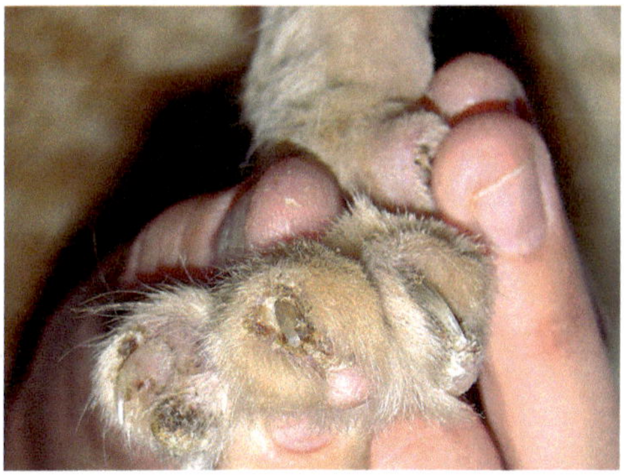

Figures 72.3. Crusted exudate around the patient's nails.

Answers Case 72

1 What pathologies should be included in the differential diagnosis of this case?

In cats, exudative and crusted lesions involving the facial area, muzzle, and nail bed are indicative of possible pemphigus foliaceus or dermatophytosis. While notoedric mange also produces crusted lesions on the face, the causative mite is easily detectable in skin scrapings and responds well to acaricidal treatment. Other less likely differential diagnoses include mosquito bite hypersensitivity and neoplasms such as epitheliotropic lymphoma.

The most probable diagnosis in this case is pemphigus foliaceus, since the exudative condition predominates and the crusted lesions around the nails and nipples are highly characteristic of this autoimmune disease. Another typical characteristic of pemphigus foliaceus in cats is the appearance of crusts on the footpads (Fig. 72.4). Although dermatophytosis is unlikely, cultures for dermatophytes should be performed to rule out infection, since the clinical appearance can be very similar.

2 What diagnostic tests should be performed?

Cytology of the lesions should be performed, especially if intact pustular lesions appear. In cases of pemphigus foliaceus, a cellular population consisting of neutrophils without toxic changes and acantholytic cells will be observed.

In this case, a biopsy revealed subcorneal pustules containing neutrophils, acantholytic cells, and eosinophils, a profile compatible with pemphigus foliaceus (Fig. 72.5).

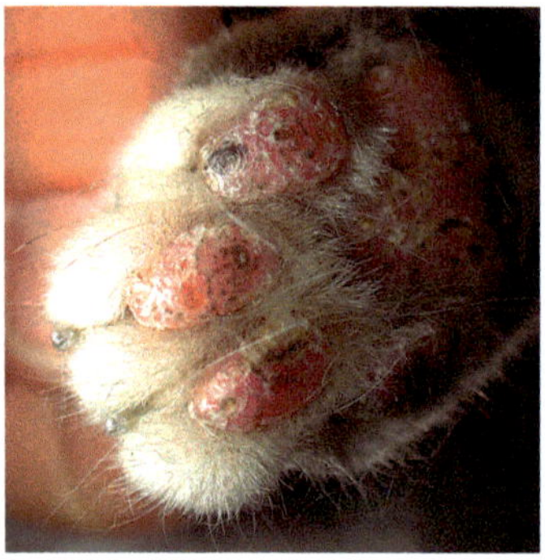

Figure 72.4. Crusted lesions on the footpads of a cat with pemphigus foliaceus.

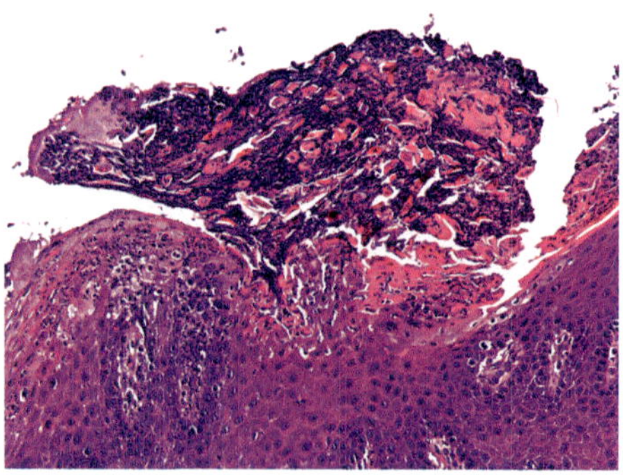

Figure 72.5. Histological examination of the patient's skin showing neutrophils, acantholytic cells, and eosinophils in both the subcorneal pustules and the crusts on the surface of the skin.

Case 73

Case presentation

The owners of a castrated male orange Tabby cat, aged 1 year, became very worried by the presence of moles on the cat's eyelid and nose.

The general condition of the cat was good. Small areas of hyperpigmentation on the eyelids and muzzle were observed in the dermatological examination (Fig. 73.1).

Questions

1. What is this alteration called?
2. What are its characteristics?

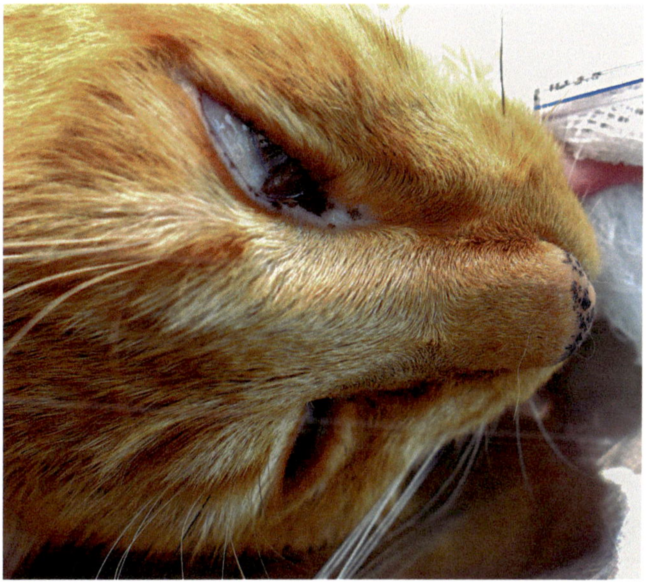

Figure 73.1. Hyperpigmented macules on the eyelids and muzzle of the patient.

Answers Case 73

1 What is this alteration called?

This condition is known as lentigo simplex, which is a hereditary pigmentary condition that is very common in cats with an orange and yellow coat. It is characterised by the appearance with age of multiple areas of black pigmentation (lentigines or hyperpigmented macules) on the gums, lips, and muzzle.

Lentigines may also appear in dogs, especially on the skin of the abdomen and on the pinnae (Fig. 73.2).

2 What are its characteristics?

Lentigo simplex is the only hereditary form of hypermelanosis described in small animals. It is an aesthetic problem, and does not require treatment.

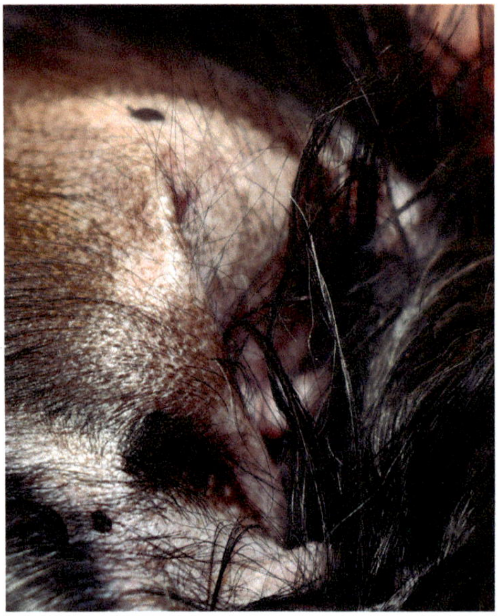

Figure 73.2. Lentigines on the pinna of a dog.

Case 74

Case presentation

Four feline patients presented with the lesions shown in Figures 74.1–74.4.

Questions

1 To which condition does each of these patterns correspond?

2 What do they have in common?

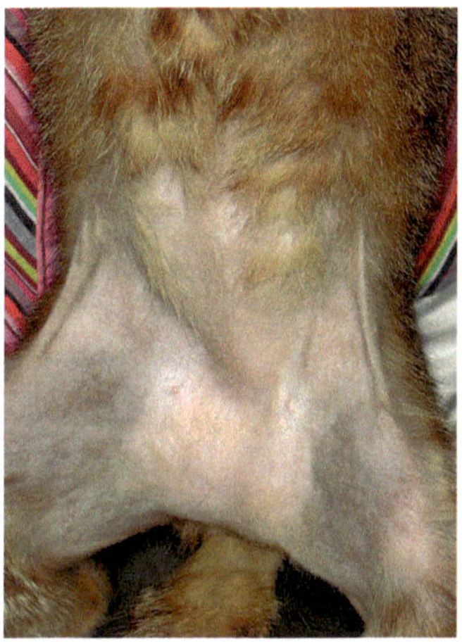

Figure 74.1.

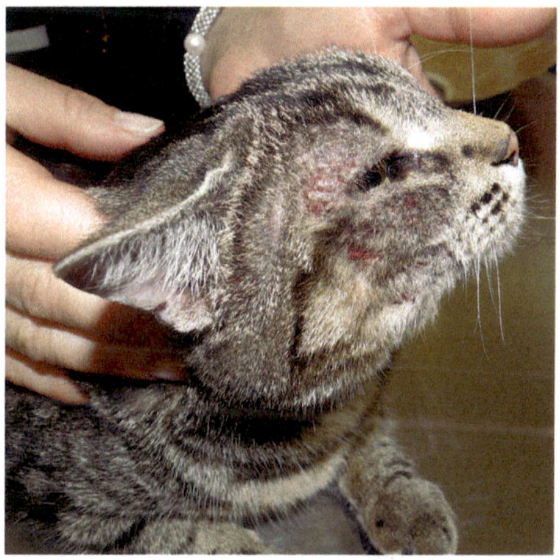

Figure 74.2.

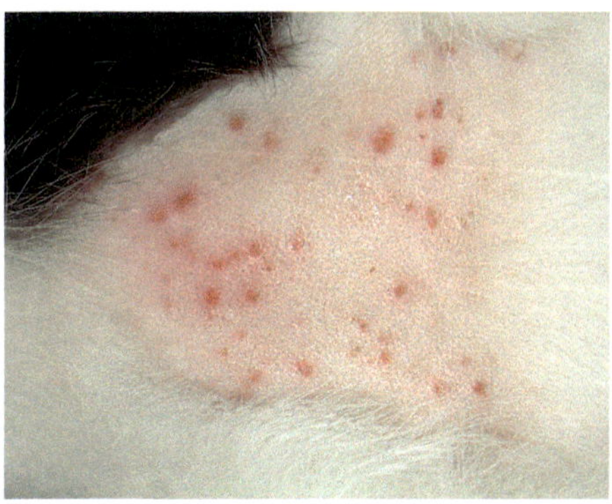

Figure 74.3.

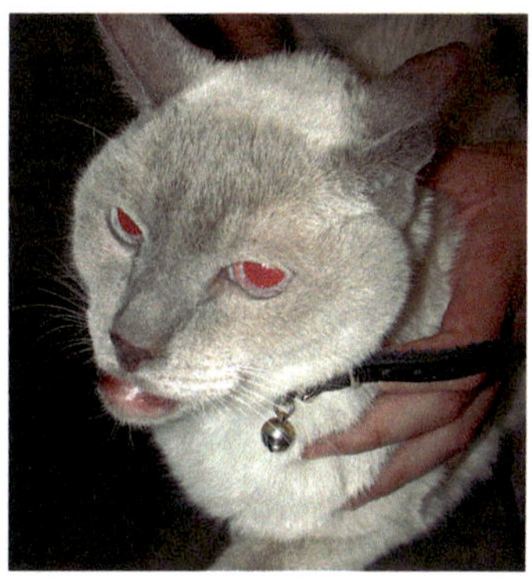

Figure 74.4.

Answers Case 74

1 To which condition does each of these patterns correspond?

Figure 74.1 corresponds to self-induced alopecia. Figure 74.2 shows a cat with pruritus of the head and neck. Figure 74.3 shows a cat with crusted papular skin lesions on the abdomen corresponding to miliary dermatitis. Figure 74.4 shows a cat with a granuloma on the chin that corresponds to eosinophilic granuloma complex.

2 What do they have in common?

All these patterns are inflammatory responses of the cat's skin to different stimuli, including hypersensitivity (food, environmental allergens, flea saliva, mosquito bites), ectoparasites (cheyletiellosis, ear mites, feline mange, demodicosis), and viral, bacterial, or fungal infections.

Self-induced alopecia in cats is usually the result of pruritus (the cat bites, scratches, or grooms excessively). The hair is broken and cannot be easily plucked out. It usually affects the skin of the abdomen, thoracolumbar area, and limbs (Fig. 74.5).

Pruritus of the face and neck is a complex syndrome caused by the same factors listed above. The pruritus is usually intense and the cat self-injures, resulting in excoriations and crusts.

Miliary dermatitis is characterised by the presence of small focal crusts that are difficult to appreciate owing to the presence of hair.

Eosinophilic granuloma complex of cats includes linear granuloma, which can affect the caudal aspect of the thighs, chin, lower lip, and oral cavity. This is usually characterised by prominent linear or nodular plaques, which can be firm or oedematous. These plaques present with mild erythema and alopecia, and may be eroded or ulcerated. Other clinical forms of feline eosinophilic granuloma complex include eosinophilic plaques and indolent ulcers (Fig. 74.6). The complex is also associated with hypersensitivity processes and bacterial infections, but in some cases can be idiopathic.

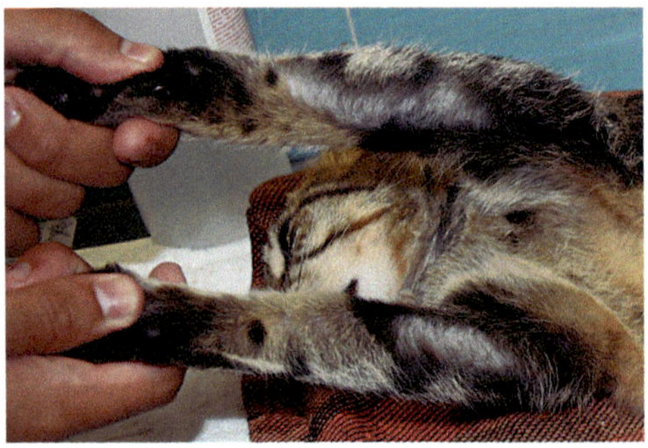

Figure 74.5. Self-induced alopecia on the inner aspect of the limbs of a cat.

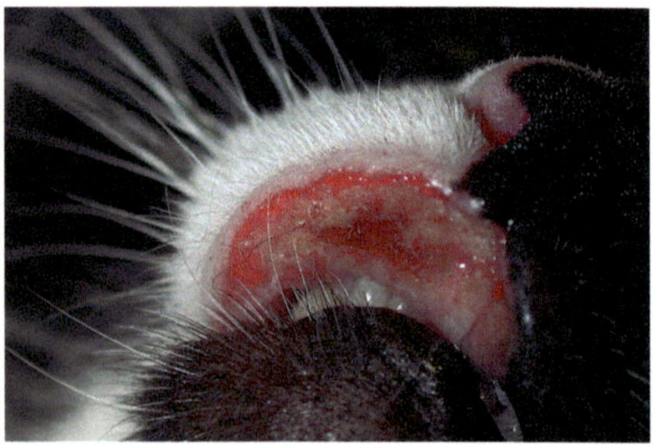

Figure 74.6. Indolent ulcer on the upper lip of a cat.

Case 75

Case presentation

The patient was an intact male Golden Retriever of 4 years of age, who had a lesion on the muzzle (Figs. 75.1 and 75.2).

Questions

1. What dermatological alteration does this patient have, and what is the most probable cause?
2. What is the physiological mechanism underlying this process?

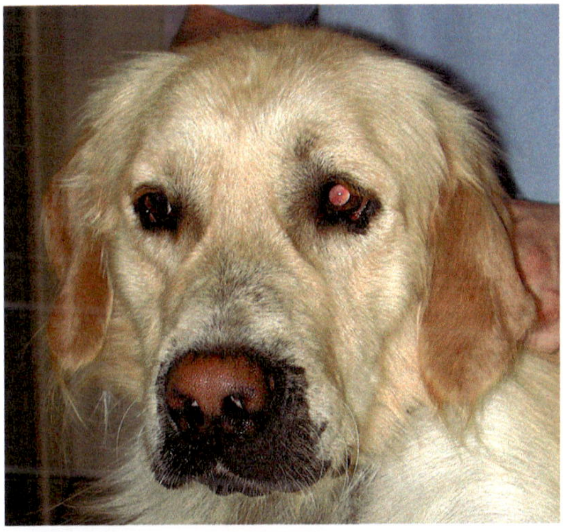

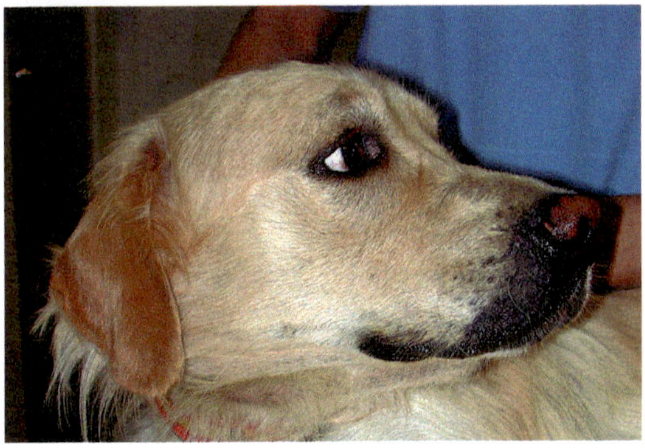

Figures 75.1 and 75.2. Lesion on the patient's muzzle.

Answers Case 75

1 What dermatological alteration does this patient have, and what is the most probable cause?

The dog has hyperpigmentation of the skin, also known as melanoderma. When hyperpigmentation affects the hair, it is called melanotrichia. In dogs, severe inflammatory processes are the most common cause of acquired noninflammatory hyperpigmentation of the skin. In this case the owners confirmed that the dog had had severe neutrophilic vasculitis of the skin 3 months earlier. Postinflammatory hyperpigmentation can be focal or circumscribed, with a patchy, diffuse, or reticular pattern (Fig. 75.3). The exact mechanism by which this hyperpigmentation occurs is unknown. Lentigo and melanoma should also be included in the differential diagnosis.

2 What is the physiological mechanism underlying this process?

Melanin, the skin's physiological pigment, is produced by melanocytes, which are located in the basal layer of the epidermis and the hair follicle. Melanin is formed in the melanosome, a specialised organelle of the melanocyte. Melanocytes transfer melanin to keratinocytes via a process known as cytocrinia. The colour of the skin is determined by the size, number, type, and distribution of the melanosomes. Melanocytes are also found in the dermis, but do not transfer melanin to the keratinocytes.

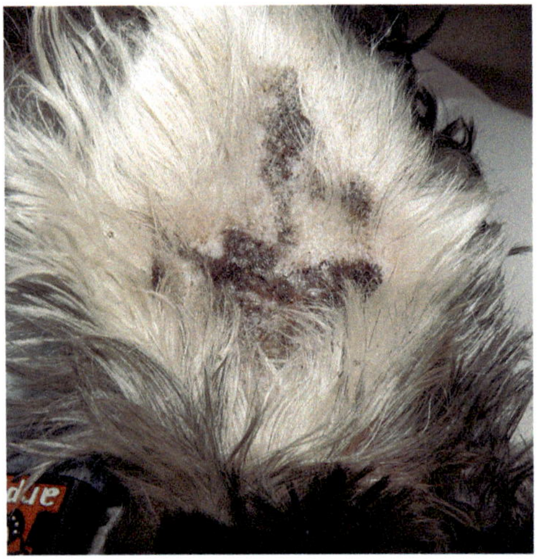

Figure 75.3. Localised postinflammatory hyperpigmentation in a reticular pattern on the inner aspect of a dog's pinna.

Case 76

Case presentation

The patient was 4-month-old male mongrel puppy with a clinical history of skin problems that had begun 1 month prior to consultation. Clinical signs had appeared 10 days after the dog had received a booster dose of the hexavalent vaccine. The owners had observed inflammation and redness that initially affected the area around the eyes and later progressed to the muzzle and chin. The lesions appeared to irritate the dog, who attempted to touch and scratch his face. He also appeared to be apathetic and lethargic. His usual veterinary surgeon had prescribed antibiotics for 10 days, with no improvement.

Moderate enlargement of all the peripheral lymph nodes was observed in the general examination. The dermatological examination revealed alopecia and erythema of the eyelids, with mild oedema, and alopecia, oedema, and swelling of the muzzle and lips (Figs. 76.1 and 76.2). Erythema was also observed on the inner aspect of the pinnae (Fig. 76.3).

Questions

1 What are the relevant differential diagnoses in this case?

2 What diagnostic tests should be performed?

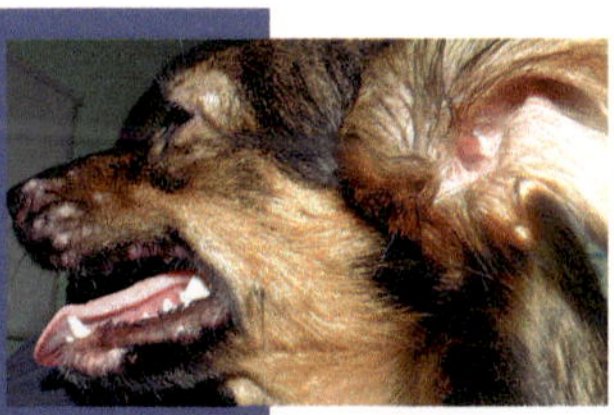

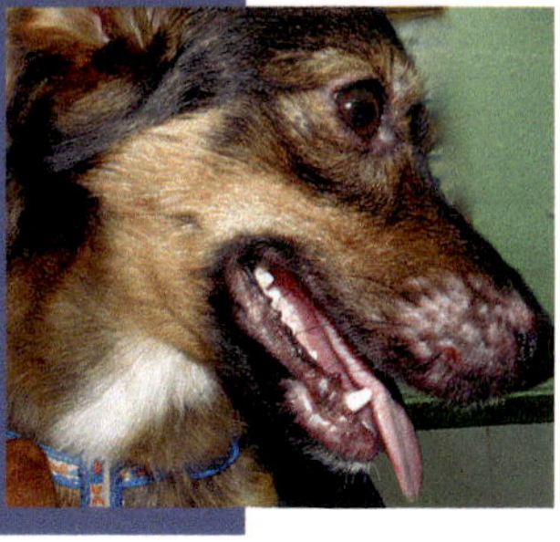

Figures 76.1 and 76.2. Erythema, alopecia, oedema, and swelling of eyelids, muzzle, and lips.

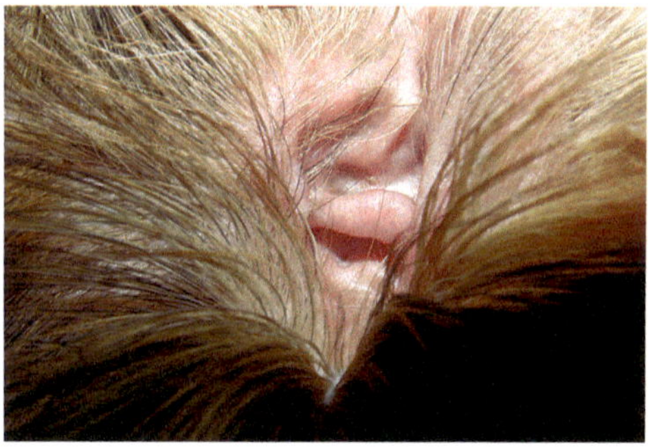

Figure 76.3. Erythema on the inner aspect of the pinna.

Answers Case 76

1 What are the relevant differential diagnoses in this case?

The following are the most likely differential diagnoses for this clinical picture:

- Generalised demodicosis.
- Juvenile cellulitis.
- Angioedema.
- Distemper.
- Deep pyoderma.
- Dermatophytosis.

2 What diagnostic tests should be performed?

Multiple tests are indicated, including skin scrapings to rule out *Demodex,* exudate cytology, fine-needle aspiration of the lymph nodes, and cultures for bacteria and dermatophytes. In this case, the tests were negative for infectious and parasitic agents. A biopsy revealed pyogranulomatous dermatitis with panniculitis that was compatible with juvenile cellulitis.

Juvenile cellulitis is an immune-mediated disease of unknown aetiology. It is treated with immunosuppressive doses of glucocorticoids that can be combined with cyclosporine. In very severe cases it can cause fibrosis and the formation of permanent scar tissue (Fig. 76.4).

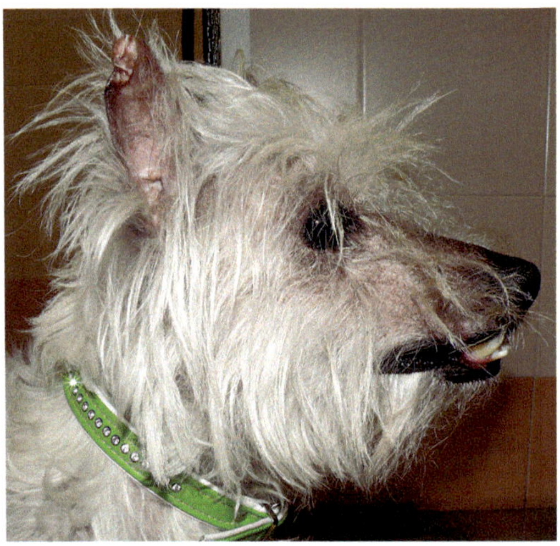

Figure 76.4. Dog with scarring alopecia secondary to juvenile cellulitis.

Case 77

Case presentation

A spayed female domestic shorthair cat, aged 13 years, was brought to the clinic for follow-up of a surgical intervention for a herniated disc (L7–S1) performed 1 week earlier. The appearance of the skin around the suture is shown in Figure 77.1. The cat displayed pain on palpation.

Questions

1. What type of lesion is this?
2. What are the possible causes?

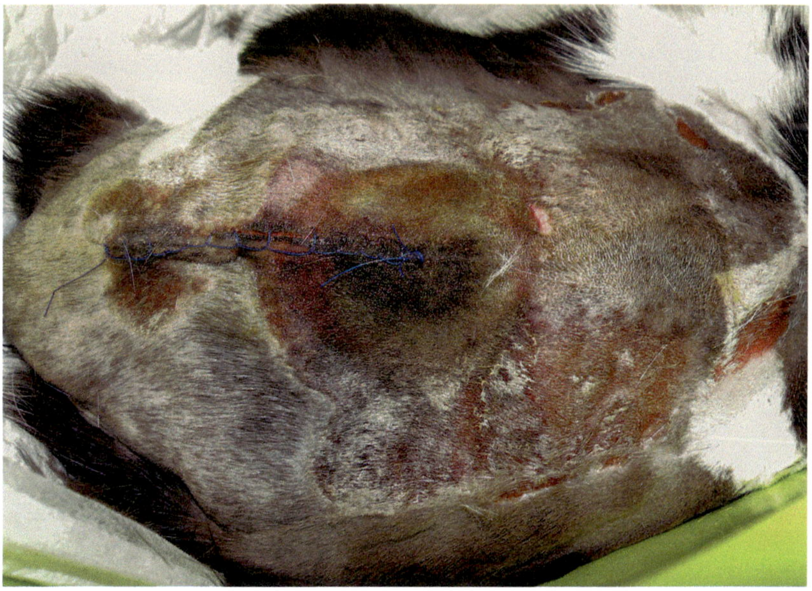

Figure 77.1. Lesion around the suture.

Answers Case 77

1 What type of lesion is this?

This lesion is known as an eschar. This is a generic term used to describe the presence of necrotic tissue on the skin surface or in subcutaneous tissue or mucous membranes.

2 What are the possible causes?

Eschar is usually secondary to skin trauma that results in a lack of vascularisation and secondary necrosis. Heat sources are the most common cause. In this clinical case, the scarification of the skin may be the result of cold applied to the area after surgery to reduce inflammation and pain. Other potential causes include the use of aggressive topical medications, injections, drug reactions, and physical trauma such as that caused by a blow or dragging.

Treatment in patients with widespread and deep eschar consists of surgical debridement of the necrotic tissue, keeping the adjacent skin in the best possible state.

Case 78

Case presentation

Skin lesions appeared abruptly in two dogs (Figs. 78.1 and 78.2).

Questions

1. What lesions are these?
2. What could have caused them?

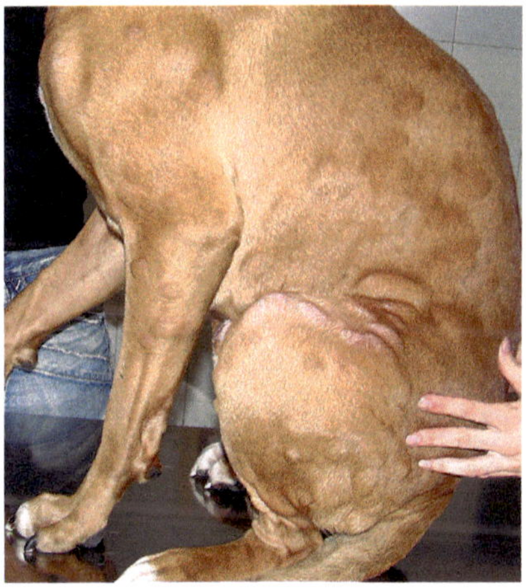

Figure 78.1. Boxer with acute generalised lesions.

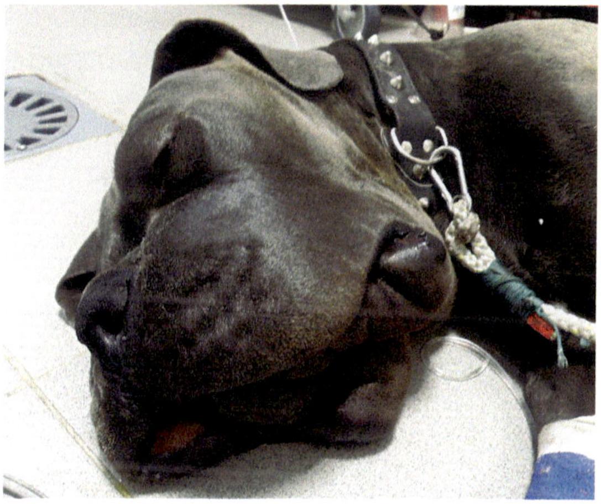

Figure 78.2. Appearance of the facial area of a Dogue de Bordeaux.

Answers Case 78

1 What lesions are these?

The dog in Figure 78.1 has multiple wheals and the patient in Figure 78.2 has facial angioedema. A wheal is a localised oedema in the superficial dermis (Fig. 78.3). Angioedema is caused by oedema and diffuse inflammation in the deep dermis or the hypodermis. Urticaria is a pathology characterised by the presence of wheals and/or angioedema. Wheals can appear anywhere on the body, while angioedema usually affects the head or the distal portion of the limbs (Fig. 78.4). Pruritus may or may not be present. Urticaria is a cutaneous clinical sign typical of an anaphylactic reaction, and may or may not be accompanied by other systemic clinical signs.

2 What could have caused them?

Anaphylaxis is a severe hypersensitivity response of hyperacute onset (within minutes or hours) that can be life threatening. In dogs, anaphylaxis is usually accompanied by gastrointestinal (vomiting and diarrhoea) or cardiovascular (vasodilatation of the hepatic artery and increased venous resistance of the liver) clinical signs. In urticaria and anaphylaxis, the activation of mast cells and basophils triggers the release of cytokines, which cause vasodilation, plasma extravasation, and activation of sensory nerve fibres. The most common causes of this type of reaction in dogs are food, biting and sucking insects, and drugs.

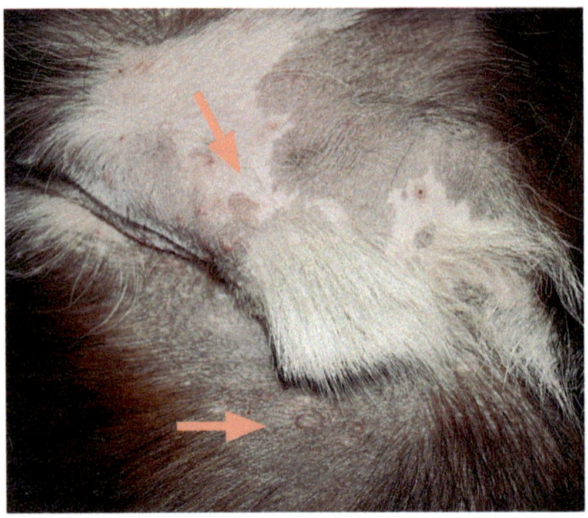

Figure 78.3. The arrows indicate the presence of wheals on the skin of the dog's abdomen caused by contact with nettles.

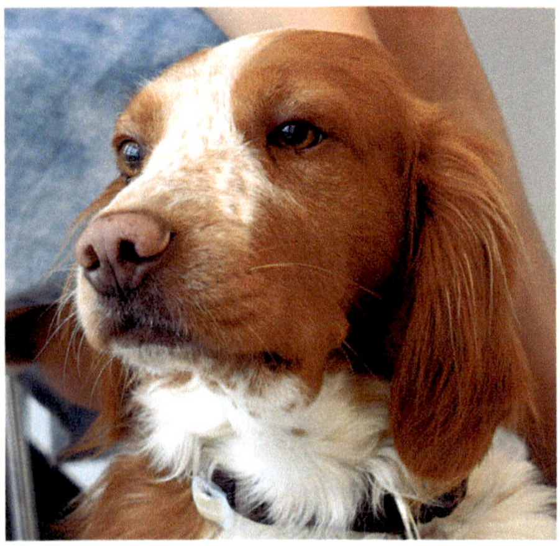

Figure 78.4. Facial angioedema.

Case 79

Case presentation

An 8-year-old intact male German Wirehaired Pointer was brought to the veterinary clinic by his owners, who reported that he had injuries on his legs. The dog licked continuously. He had been treated with antibiotics and nonsteroidal anti-inflammatory drugs, with no improvement. His general condition was good. He usually went hunting with his owner.

He had an ulcerated nodular lesion on the skin of the lower portion of the right hock. In the axillary area of the right forelimb, nodules and plaques that drained a haemorrhagic exudate were detected (Figs. 79.1 and 79.2). Cytology of the exudate was performed (Figs. 79.3–79.5).

Questions

1 What does the cytology reveal?

2 Taking into account the clinical history, the appearance of the lesions, and the cytological profile, what is the most likely diagnosis?

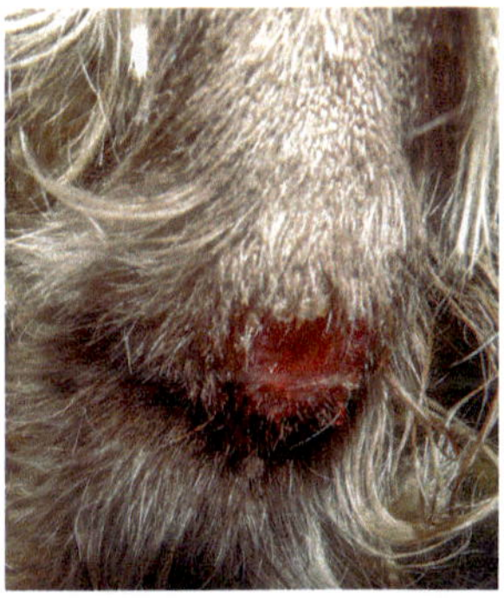

Figure 79.1. Ulcerated lesion on the skin beneath the patient's hock.

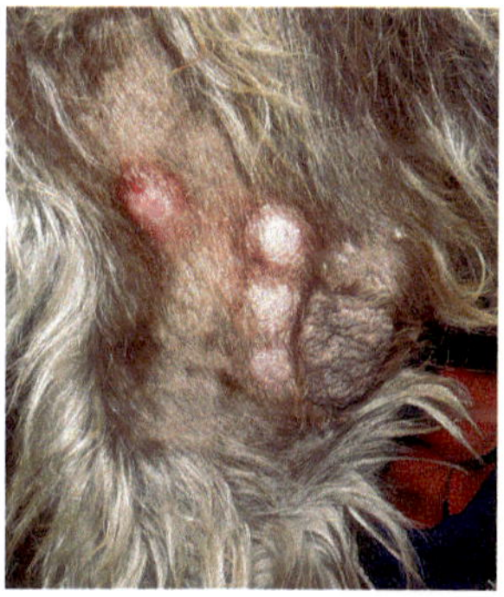

Figure 79.2. Nodules and plaques with haemorrhagic exudate on the medial aspect of the limb.

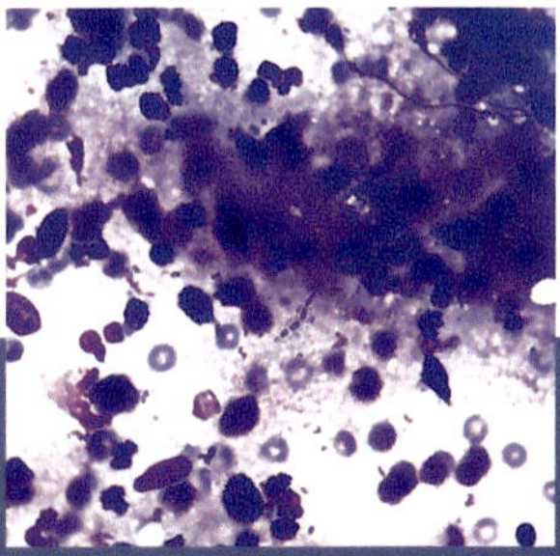

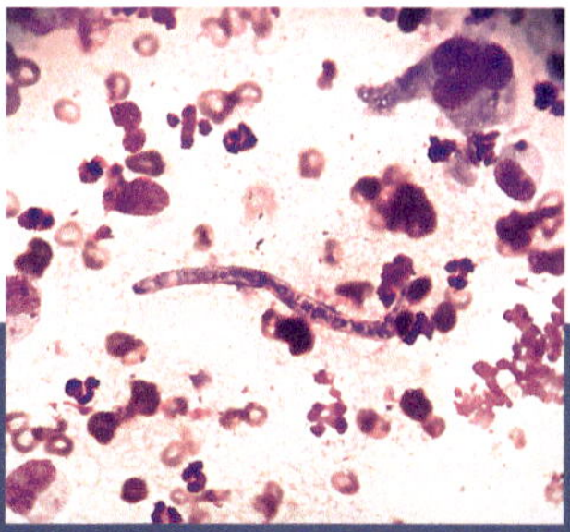

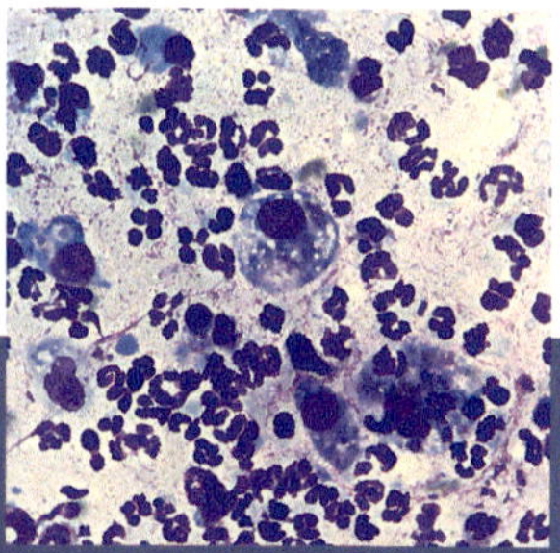

Figures 79.3–79.5. Cytology of lesion exudate.

Answers Case 79

1 What does the cytology reveal?

Cytology shows a cell population consisting of neutrophilic granulocytes and macrophages. Arthrospores and fungal hyphae are also evident.

2 Taking into account the clinical history, the appearance of the lesions, and the cytological profile, what is the most likely diagnosis?

Dermatophytic kerion, mycetoma, and phaeohyphomycosis should be included in the differential diagnosis of a cutaneous nodule with a pyogranulomatous inflammatory process and the presence of arthrospores and fungal hyphae. A kerion is an inflammatory response to a dermatophyte, most commonly *Microsporum gypseum* and *Trichophyton mentagrophytes*. A mycetoma is a subcutaneous granulomatous infection that can be caused by fungi or bacteria such as *Actinomyces* or *Nocardia*. Phaeohyphomycosis is a subcutaneous infection caused by pigmented or opportunistic fungi.

In this case, the culture was positive for *Trichophyton mentagrophytes* (Fig. 79.6). This fungus is associated with the presence of rodents, horses, and cows.

The patient was treated with oral itraconazole, resulting in resolution of the lesions after 5 weeks (Fig. 79.7).

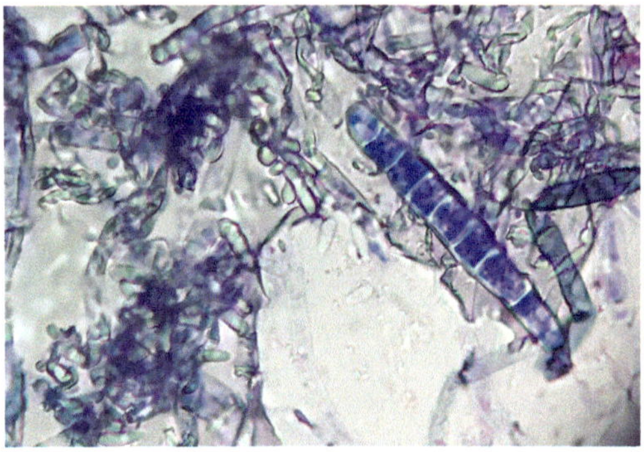

Figure 79.6. Macroconidium of *Trichophyton mentagrophytes*.

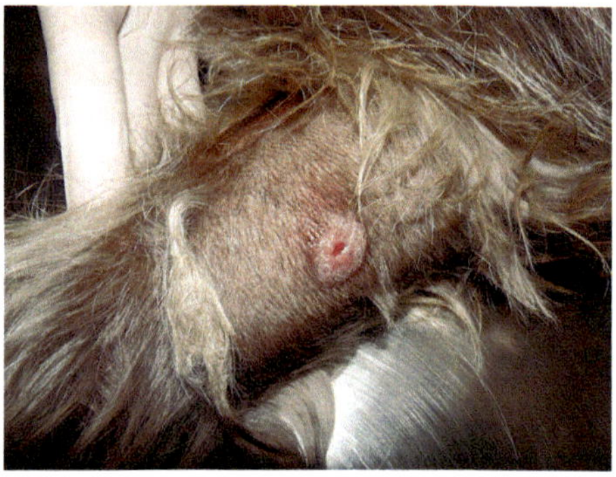

Figure 79.7. Appearance of a nodule 3 weeks after starting treatment with itraconazole.

Case 80

Case presentation

The patient was a Basset Hound who was predisposed to otitis externa (OE) (Fig. 80.1).

Questions

1. What factors predispose dogs to otitis externa?
2. What are the primary causes of otitis externa in dogs and cats?

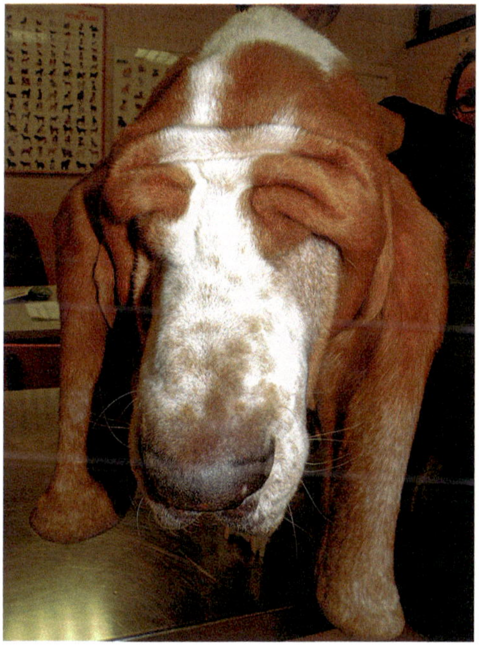

Figure 80.1. Basset Hound.

Answers Case 80

1 What factors predispose dogs to otitis externa?

Ear conformation is one of the factors that predisposes animals to OE. In dogs with pendulous ears, such as the Basset Hound, aeration of the ear canal is restricted, favouring the development of secondary infections. Other aspects of the ear conformation that predispose dogs to OE include narrow or hairy ear canals and ear canal atresia, as found in Shar Peis (Fig. 80.2). Excessive cerumen production, increased humidity caused by excessive cleaning or bathing, and the use of aggressive cleaning techniques can predispose dogs to OE.

2 What are the primary causes of otitis externa in dogs and cats?

The following are the primary causes of OE:

- Parasites (*Otodectes cynotis*, *Demodex*).
- Foreign bodies.
- Hypersensitivity (atopy, food and contact allergy).
- Primary seborrhoeic disorders.
- Immune-mediated diseases.
- Endocrine diseases (hypothyroidism).
- Inflammatory polyps.
- Neoplasms (sebaceous gland adenocarcinoma, basal cell carcinoma, squamous cell carcinoma).
- Idiopathic hyperplasia of the ceruminous and sebaceous glands.

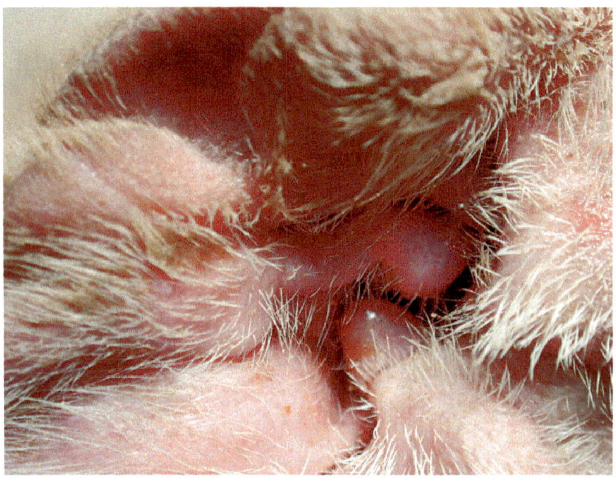

Figure 80.2. Ear canal stenosis in a Shar Pei.

Case 81

Case presentation

The owners of an intact male Beagle, aged 1 year, reported that he had lost hair from the eyelid and sternum, and that his skin was irritated and itchy. Four months earlier he had been diagnosed with immune-mediated meningitis and had since been treated with glucocorticoids (2.5 mg of prednisone every 24 hours). The dog weighed 18 kg. The owners had also observed that the hair on the back of the neck had not grown back after clipping prior to the extraction of cerebrospinal fluid.

The results of the general examination were normal. Alopecia with erythema was observed on the eyelid, alopecia on the sternum, and hypotrichosis in the clipped area on the back of the neck (Figs. 81.1–81.3).

Questions

1 Is the alopecia presented by this patient inflammatory or noninflammatory?

2 If inflammatory, what would be the main differential diagnoses?

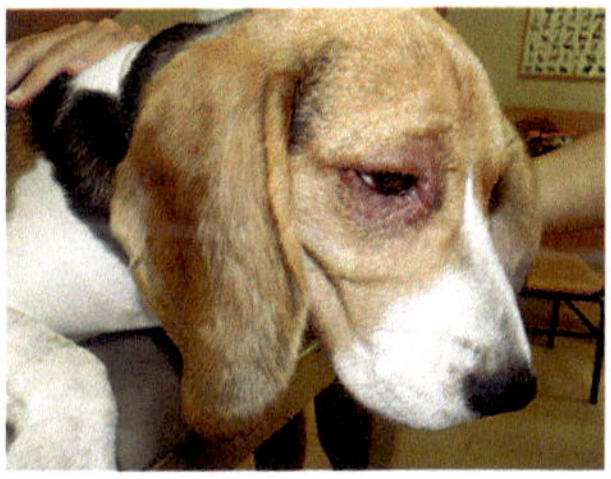

Figure 81.1. Alopecia and erythema on the patient's eyelid.

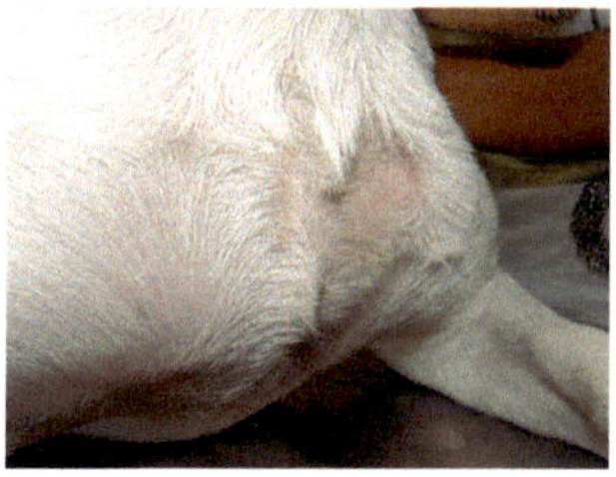

Figure 81.2. Focal alopecia in the area of the sternum.

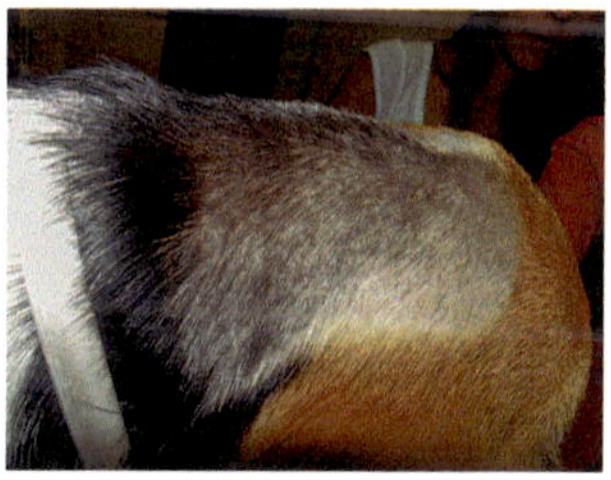

Figure 81.3. Hypotrichosis in the dorsal area of the neck.

Answers Case 81

1 Is the alopecia presented by this patient inflammatory or noninflammatory?

The alopecia affecting the eyelid and sternum appears to be inflammatory, since it is associated with erythema and pruritus.

2 If inflammatory, what would be the main differential diagnoses?

Demodicosis, dermatophytosis, and bacterial folliculitis are among the most likely differential diagnoses in a young dog undergoing chronic glucocorticoid treatment. Numerous *Demodex canis* mites were evident in the patient's trichogram (Fig. 81.4).

In the dorsal area, the hypotrichosis appears to be noninflammatory and is highly localised, limited to the clipped area. The most probable diagnosis is post-clipping alopecia. This is an idiopathic disorder, and does not require treatment. The aetiology is unknown but appears to involve an interruption of the follicular cycle. Hair can take up to 24 months to grow. Glucocorticoids are also inhibitors of the follicular cycle and can contribute to the persistence of alopecia.

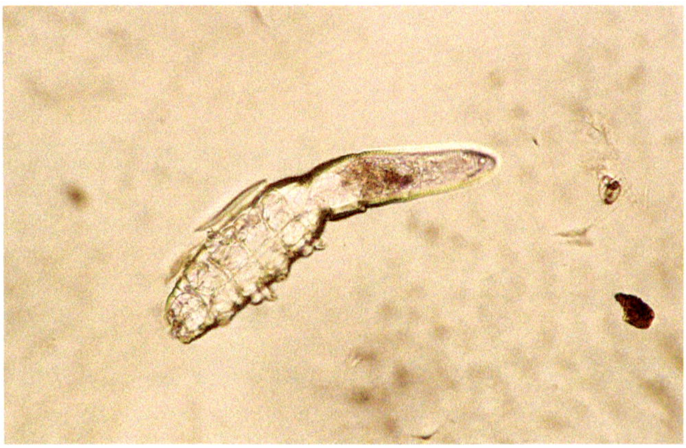

Figure 81.4. Adult *Demodex canis* mite.

Case 82

Case presentation

A castrated male domestic shorthair cat, aged 10 years, was brought for consultation with multiple nodules on the head, neck, and skin of the abdomen. The lesions were not pruritic and the cat was in good health. His owner was a missionary who had lived together with the cat in Israel during the First Gulf War.

The results of the general examination and blood tests were normal. The lesions were raised, rounded, well-defined masses of variable size that adhered to the surrounding skin (Figs. 82.1–82.3). Aspiration cytology of the nodules and tumours showed multiple round cells of variable size with anisokaryosis, as well as multinucleated cells. The cells had a histiocytic appearance, with no granules evident in the cytoplasm (Fig. 82.4).

Questions

1. What are the possible diagnoses based on the clinical appearance of the lesions and the cytological profile?
2. What other tests could we perform to confirm the diagnosis?

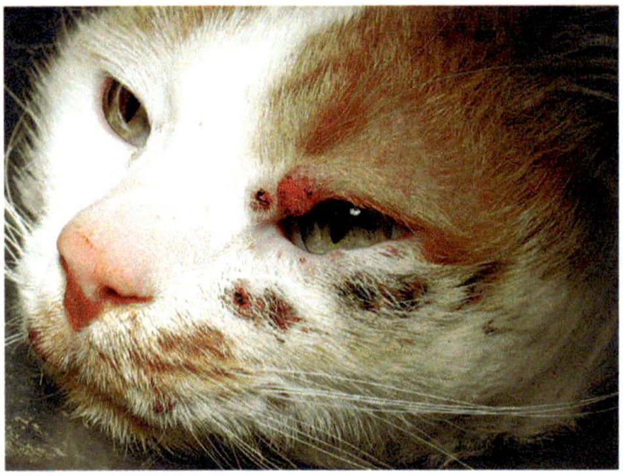

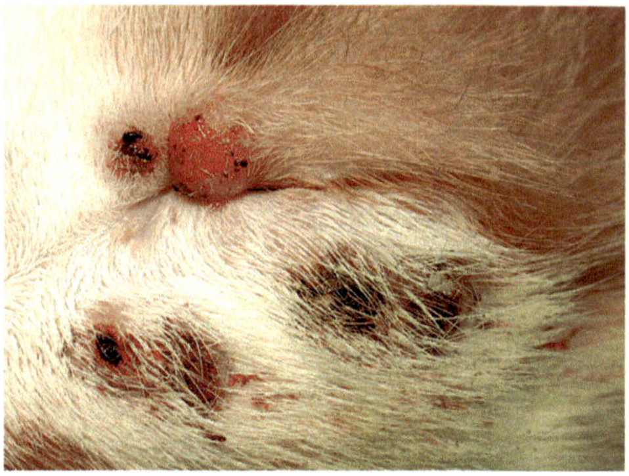

Figures 82.1 and 82.2. Multiple nodules, some ulcerated and crusted, on the face and eyelid of the patient.

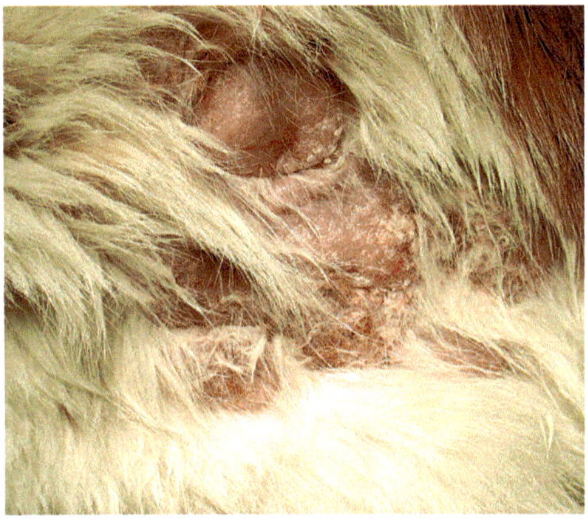

Figure 82.3. Masses on the skin of the abdomen.

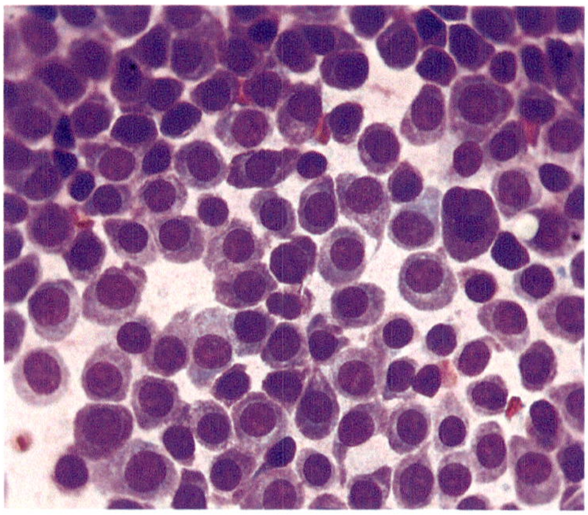

Figure 82.4. Cytological image of the lesions.

Answers Case 82

1 What are the possible diagnoses based on the clinical appearance of the lesions and the cytological profile?

Multiple nodules together with suspicion of a round cell neoplasm are strongly suggestive of cutaneous mast cell tumours. Other differential diagnoses include epitheliotropic lymphoma and histiocytic mast cell tumours.

2 What other tests could we perform to confirm the diagnosis?

To confirm the diagnosis, a biopsy of the nodules was performed. The histological examination revealed an infiltrate containing markedly pleomorphic round cells with a high mitotic index (2–3 mitoses per field). The cells contained moderate amounts of eosinophilic cytoplasmic granules and a central nucleus with compact chromatin. Staining with toluidine blue revealed occasional metachromatic cytoplasmic granules in the neoplastic cells. In immunohistochemical analyses the sample was positive for the oncological marker c-kit (CD117). A definitive diagnosis of high-grade mastocytoma was established. Thoracic radiographs and abdominal ultrasound revealed no findings of note.

Observations

Mast cell tumours in cats have three clinical forms:

- Cutaneous: limited to the skin.
- Lymphoreticular or visceral: can affect the liver, spleen, or abdominal lymph nodes.
- Gastrointestinal: the digestive form behaves like a primary tumour and its incidence is high, albeit lower than that of intestinal lymphoma and adenocarcinoma.

Cutaneous mast cell tumours can be histiocytic or mastocytic. Solitary, low-grade mast cell tumours with no lymph node involvement have a good prognosis (Fig. 82.5). Survival time in cats with multiple, poorly differentiated tumours and nodal or splenic involvement is much lower.

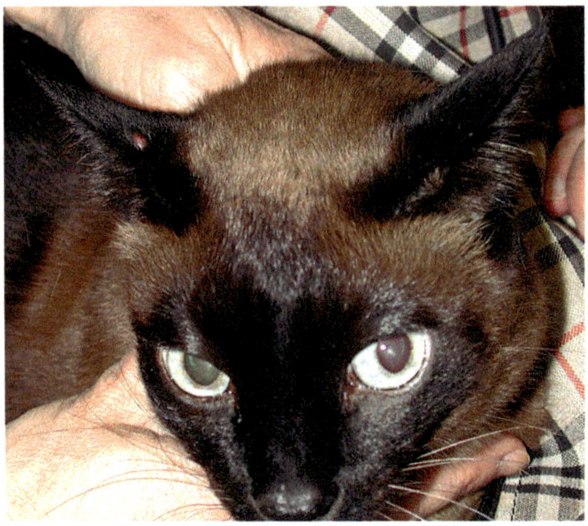

Figure 82.5. Solitary mastocytoma on the pinna of a Siamese cat.

Case 83

Case presentation

The owner of a 7-year-old male mongrel dog reported that 2 months earlier he had detected lesions on both his dog's ears. These had progressively worsened (Fig. 83.1), but the dog's general condition was good.

Questions

1. What pathologies should be included in the differential diagnosis in this case?
2. What diagnostic tests would be indicated?

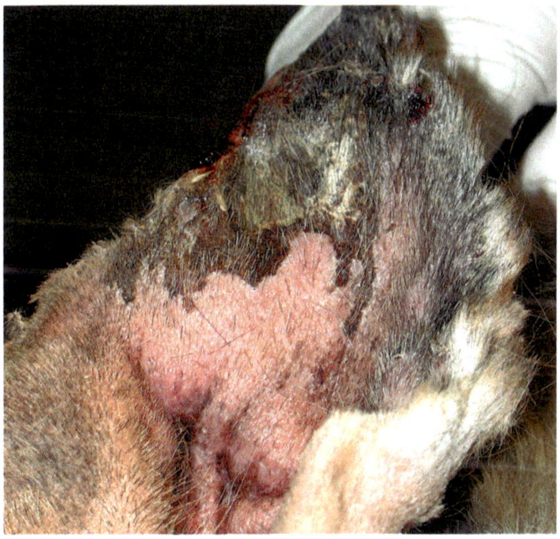

Figure 83.1. Lesions on the pinna of the patient.

Answers Case 83

1 What pathologies should be included in the differential diagnosis in this case?

The following are the most likely differential diagnoses:

- Vasculitis.
- Drug reaction.
- Ulcerative lesions caused by hyperadrenocorticism.
- Idiopathic proliferative thrombovascular necrosis of the tip of the pinna.

2 What diagnostic tests would be indicated?

Biopsy is the test that provides the most information. The pinna is a difficult location from which to obtain a biopsy. In this case it is necessary to obtain a sample with wide margins.

Proliferative thrombovascular necrosis is a disease of unknown aetiology with no reported age-, sex-, or breed-related predisposition. It manifests as small ulcers or erosions in the apical margin of the pinnae that extend across the concave surface, evolving into areas of necrosis and deforming the ears.

In this case, the patient had proliferative thrombovascular necrosis, which was treated by surgical removal of the necrotic tissue and oral administration of pentoxifylline to prevent the appearance of new lesions.

Case 84

Case presentation

An intact male Persian cat, aged 3 years, was brought to our centre with a pruritic condition that affected the facial area and had appeared 2 years earlier. His owners complained that the hair in this area had always appeared "greasy". The patient had very extensive erythematous and exudative lesions, with excoriations in the auricular and periocular areas and on the face, chin, and neck (Figs. 84.1). Bilateral ceruminous otitis externa was also evident. These same lesions, although less evident, were also present in the perianal and genital areas. The exudate was dark and very abundant. All other findings of the physical examination were normal.

The results of all basic diagnostic tests (scrapings, fungal culture, etc.) were negative. Cytology of the exudate showed polymorphonuclear neutrophils, many bacteria (cocci and bacilli), and *Malassezia* spp. The results of FeLV and FIV tests were negative, while the blood count revealed mild eosinophilia (2.2×10^9/l). The skin biopsy revealed intense epithelial hyperplasia, with foci of hyperkeratosis and parakeratosis. Exocytosis with keratin accumulation and cell debris was evident in the outermost layers. An intense inflammatory infiltrate composed of many mast cells and some lymphocytes was observed in the dermoepidermal junction. Focal areas of spongiosis appeared in the epithelium. Marked dilation and hyperplasia of the sebaceous glands was observed, and the hair follicles were surrounded by inflammatory cells (mainly neutrophils) (Fig. 84.2).

Questions

1 Taking into account the species, breed, and clinical characteristics, what is the most likely diagnosis?

2 What are the likely prognosis and appropriate treatment for this disease?

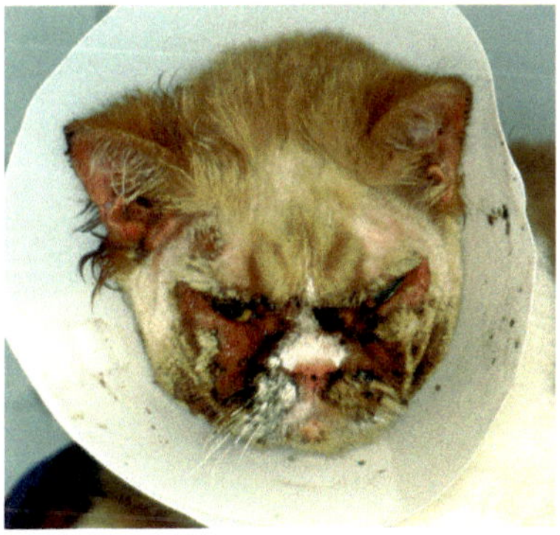

◀ Figure 84.1. Symmetric, erythematous, erosive and highly exudative lesions on the pinnae and in the periocular and perioral areas.

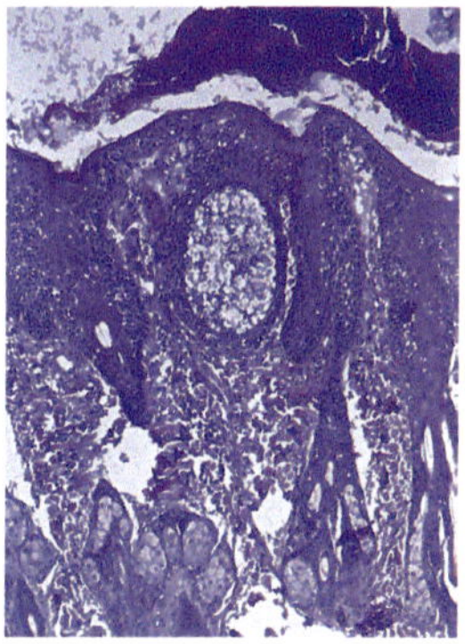

Figure 84.2. Histological image of the lesions showing acanthosis, epidermal spongiosis, serocellular crusts, and sebaceous hyperplasia. ▶

Answers Case 84

1 Taking into account the species, breed, and clinical characteristics, what is the most likely diagnosis?

The most likely diagnosis is idiopathic facial dermatitis of Persian and Himalayan cats. This form of dermatitis is characterised by the presence of a dark exudate around the eyes and mouth and on the skin of the chin. The presence of this exudate results in matted and greasy-looking hair. Affected cats usually develop bacterial infections caused by *Malassezia*, suggesting secondary infections can complicate the clinical picture in this syndrome (although partial responses to antibiotics and antifungals are observed in some cases).

While the origin of the dark exudate that adheres to the hair is unknown, it may be the result of excess production by the sebaceous glands. The cat's response to corticosteroids was variable, and generally poor, suggesting that this dermatitis is not one of the more common facial dermatoses, such as atopy or food allergy.

The cause of this dermatosis is unknown, but it appears to be due to abnormal function of the sebaceous glands, and may also involve a hereditary component.

2 What are the likely prognosis and appropriate treatment for this disease?

To date, no specific treatment for this condition has been described, although some patients may improve following the administration of oral cyclosporine or topical tacrolimus twice daily. The prognosis is reserved to poor, and many cats require a permanent Elizabethan collar to prevent self-injury (Fig. 84.3).

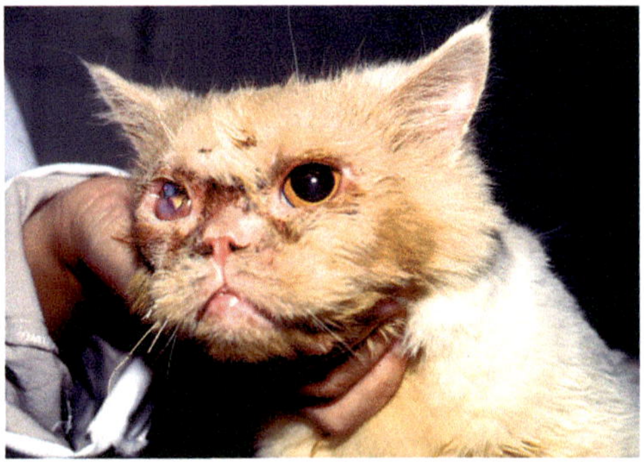

Figure 84.3. Persian cat with idiopathic facial dermatitis and a corneal ulcer caused by pruritus-induced self-injury.

Case 85

Case presentation

An intact male English Bulldog, aged 3 years, was brought for a dermatological consultation with marked pruritus of the forelimbs that had appeared 6 months earlier. The dog continuously licked between his digits, causing bleeding, and exhibited lameness. Blood allergy tests had been performed, but the results were negative. While the dog's condition had improved with oral cortisone treatment, this affected his ability to control urination, and the owners did not want to recommence this treatment.

The findings of the general examination were normal, except for moderate overweight (body condition, 5/9). Nodular violaceous lesions were observed in the dermatological examination (Figs. 85.1 and 85.2). Some of the nodules produced a haemorrhagic exudate and were painful. Cytology revealed a pyogranulomatous exudate, but no bacteria (Fig. 85.3).

Questions

1 What type of pathology is associated with this lesion, and what is it called when this location is affected?

2 What are the causes of this syndrome and what are the available therapeutic options?

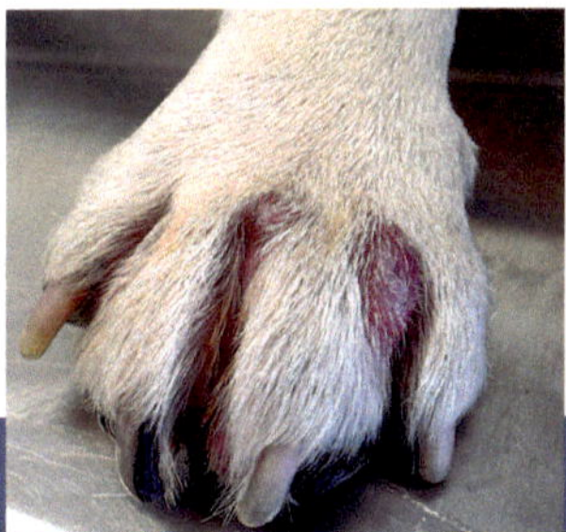

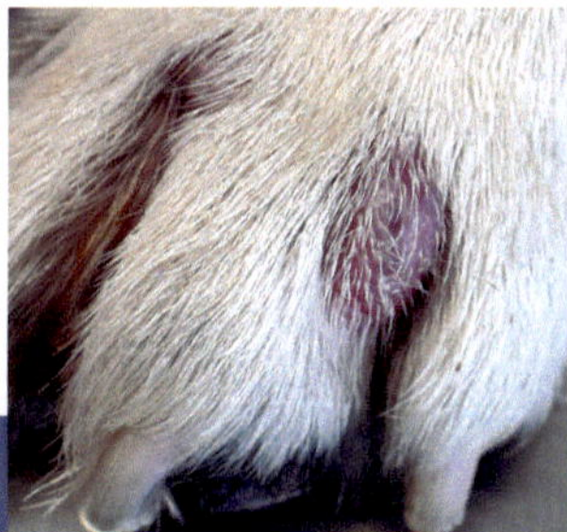

Figures 85.1 and 85.2. Interdigital violaceous nodular lesions. The skin in the centre of the lesion is about to rupture and fistulise.

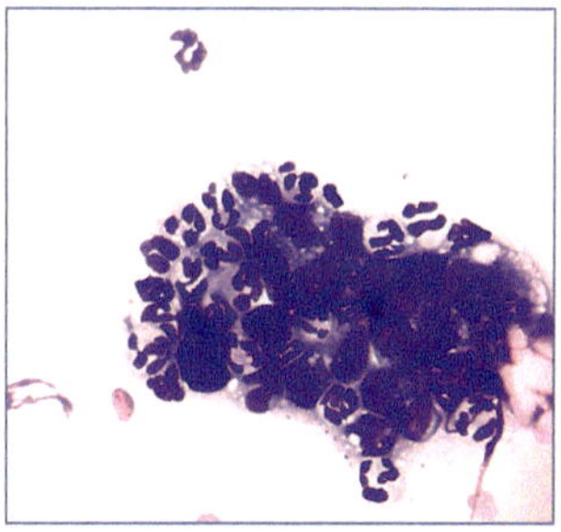

Figure 85.3. Lesion exudate composed of polymorphonuclear neutrophils and macrophages.

Answers Case 85

1 What type of pathology is associated with this lesion, and what is it called when this location is affected?

Nodular lesions with pyogranulomatous exudate suggest an inflammatory process affecting the deeper layers of the skin. This process is usually complicated by bacterial infections. When the inflammation affects the hair follicle, resulting in its rupture (folliculitis-furunculosis), the keratin of the hair acts as a foreign body and exacerbates the inflammatory process. When the nodular lesions are located in the interdigital region, the condition is described using the terms interdigital folliculitis-furunculosis, interdigital follicular cysts, or nodular pododermatitis.

The clinical signs consist of interdigital cysts, inflammation, erythema, fistulous tracts with or without haemorrhagic exudate, and ulceration (Fig. 85.4). Large muscular breeds such as the English Bulldog are predisposed to this syndrome.

2 What are the causes of this syndrome and what are the available therapeutic options?

The cause of this pathology (poor conformation and limb support, allergic factors) is unknown and the contribution of bacterial infections remains to be determined. It is recommended to rule out demodicosis and systemic infectious diseases depending on the geographical location, to perform lesion cultures and antibiograms, and to monitor the patient's weight. It is also advisable to carry out diagnostic protocols for allergic diseases if the dog has a compatible clinical picture.

Several treatments have been proposed, including the use of oral or topical antibiotics until the lesions resolve. If the patient does not respond to antibiotic treatment, administration of oral cyclosporine or immunosuppressive doses of glucocorticoids is recommended. Some authors recommend the use of surgical laser to remove the furuncles and therapeutic laser to reduce inflammation.

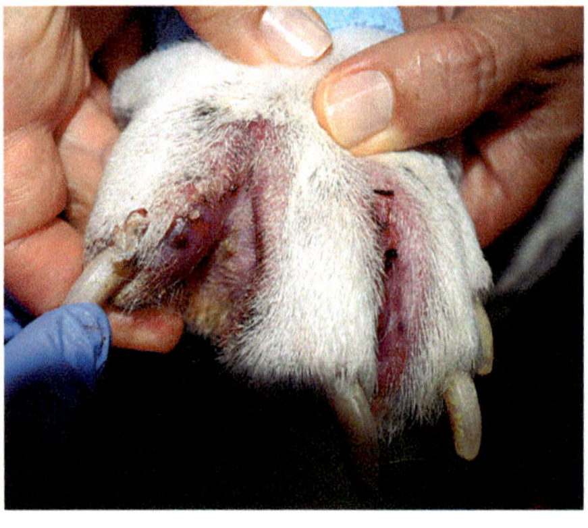

Figure 85.4. Erythema, nodules, fistulous tracts, and haemorrhagic exudate in a dog with interdigital folliculitis-furunculosis.

Case 86

Case presentation

A 6-year-old purebred male Andalusian gelding presented with intense pruritus, which provoked biting and rubbing of the affected areas against the walls of the barn. Upon examination of the haircoat, small insects were evident on the hair and the skin surface (Fig. 86.1). The parasite shown in Figure 86.2 was observed by microscopy.

Questions

1. What parasite is this?
2. How can it be treated?

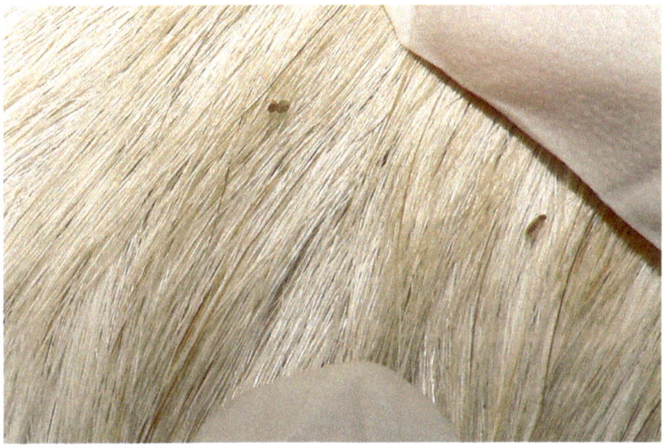

Figure 86.1. Insects on the surface of the horse skin can be observed with the naked eye.

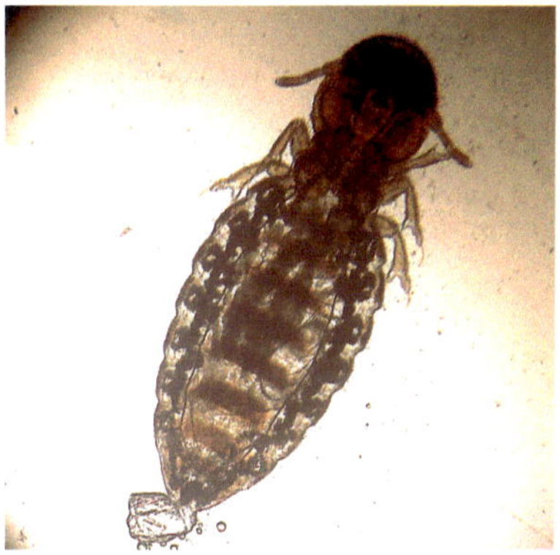

Figure 86.2. Insect as viewed under the microscope.

Answers Case 86

1 What parasite is this?

This is *Werneckiella equi equi*, a biting louse of equids found in horses stabled in poor sanitary conditions. It is usually affects horses during the winter, when animals are more closely confined.

2 How can it be treated?

The recommended treatment is ivermectin administered at 0.2 mg/kg every 14 days for 3 cycles. Permethrin (2 %), fipronil, or calcium sulfide sprays can also be administered topically every 48 hours for 3 cycles. All other horses in contact with those affected should also be treated.

Case 87

Case presentation

An intact, 3-year-old English Bulldog bitch presented with acute generalised redness of the skin. The patient had mild pruritus and her general condition was good, although her owners mentioned that she appeared slightly apathetic. Examination revealed generalised erythema mainly affecting the facial region, the inner aspects of the pinnae, the limbs, and the skin of the abdomen (Figs. 87.1 and 87.2). The macula on the skin of the abdomen was purple, and no change in colour was observed with diascopy (Figs. 87.3 and 87.4). Mild oedema of the limbs was observed. One week earlier the patient had begun oral cephalexin treatment for a superficial pyoderma. The dog's general condition deteriorated over the following 2 days, and the skin lesions acquired the appearance shown in Figure 87.5. A biopsy was performed. Histology showed keratinocyte apoptosis with lymphocyte satellitosis and mild epidermal necrosis. Oedema, microhaemorrhage, and a perivascular to interstitial inflammatory infiltrate were observed in the superficial dermis. The infiltrate consisted of mast cells, neutrophils, and lymphocytes. Fibrinoid necrosis of the subepidermal blood vessels and periadnexal vessels was evident, with the presence of intravascular thrombi and perivascular erythrocytes.

Questions

1 What types of skin lesions are seen on this patient?

2 Based on the clinical signs and histological findings, what is the most likely diagnosis?

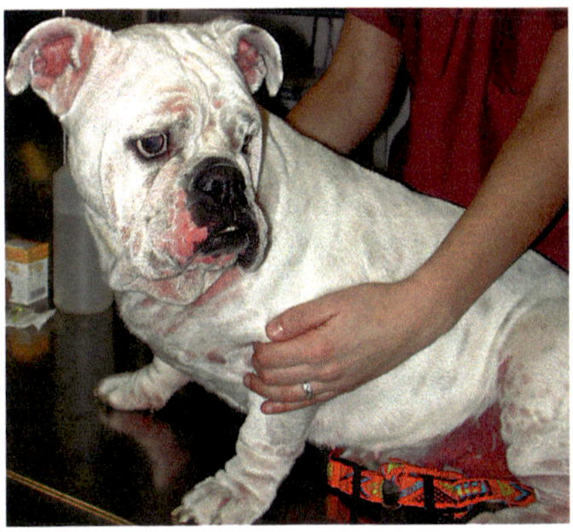

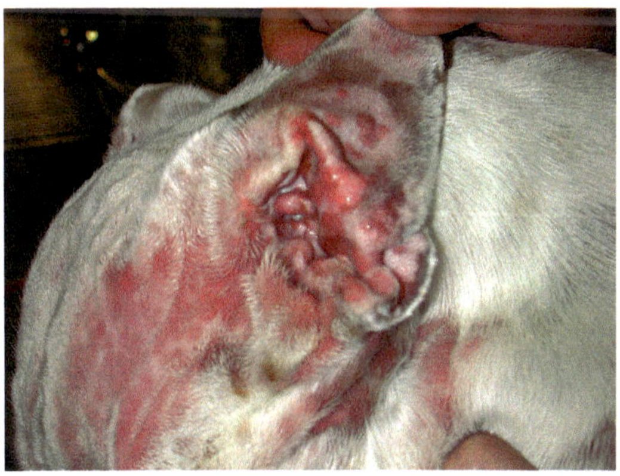

Figures 87.1 and 87.2. Generalised erythema on the face, pinnae, and trunk of the patient.

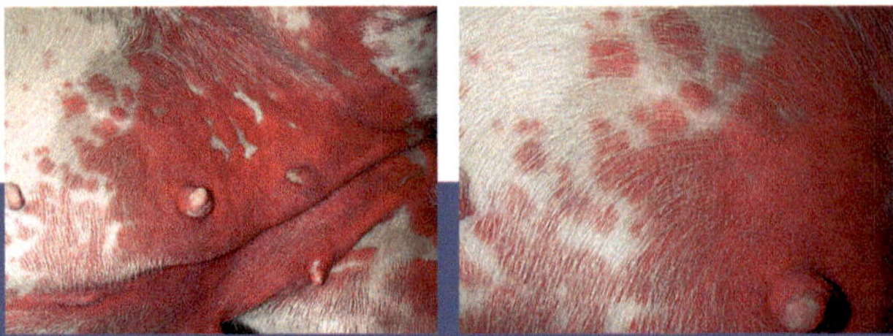

Figures 87.3 and 87.4. Erythroderma, oedema, and purpura on the skin of the abdomen.

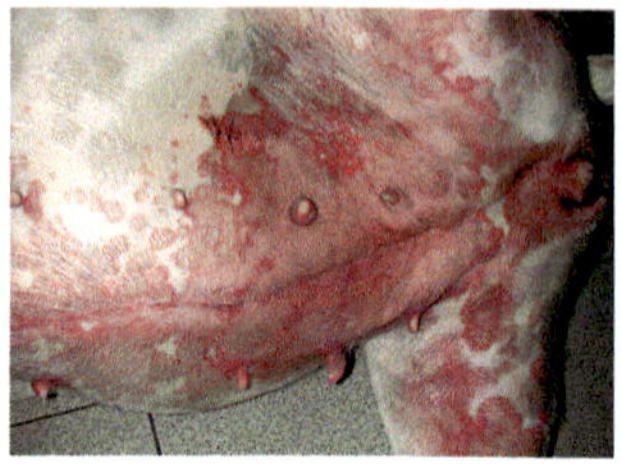

Figure 87.5. Serpiginous and target lesions on the skin of the abdomen.

Answers Case 87

1 What types of skin lesions are seen on this patient?

The patient has generalised erythroderma and oedema and purpura on the skin of the abdomen (Figs. 87.1–87.4). Two days after the initial consultation, the skin appeared less oedematous and haemorrhagic, but the patient had developed target lesions with a dark centre surrounded by a paler, erythematous halo (Fig. 87.5).

2 Based on the clinical signs and histological findings, what is the most likely diagnosis?

The clinical history, lesions, and biopsy results suggest erythema multiforme (EM) associated with vasculitis. EM is a lymphocyte-mediated disease that produces cytotoxic changes in the epidermis. In humans, EM is usually caused by infections, generally herpesviruses infections (Fig. 87.6), while in veterinary medicine it is associated with certain medications, including antibiotics (especially cephalosporins and penicillins), sulfonamides, levamisole, diethylcarbamazine, and phenobarbital.

In this case, EM may have been secondary to cephalexin administration, and the vascular inflammation associated with the drug reaction may have contributed to the oedema and initial haemorrhage.

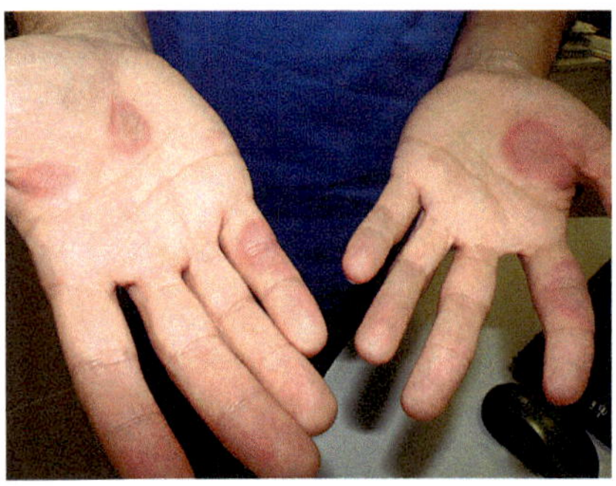

Figure 87.6. Target lesions typical of erythema multiforme in humans.

Case 88

Case presentation

An intact, 8-year-old European Shorthair cat presented with skin lesions on the abdomen that exuded pus (Fig. 88.1). The cat, which had tested negative for feline leukaemia and feline immunodeficiency virus, lived in a rural house and had access to the outdoors. Despite repeated treatments with dilute chlorhexidine, the placement of surgical drains, and repeated cefovecin injections over the preceding 2 months, the lesions had failed to heal, but had improved somewhat. The abscesses were exclusively located in the inguinal area and the cat's general condition was good.

Questions

1. What dermatological lesions does this cat have and what pathologies should be included in the differential diagnosis?
2. What diagnostic tests should be performed?

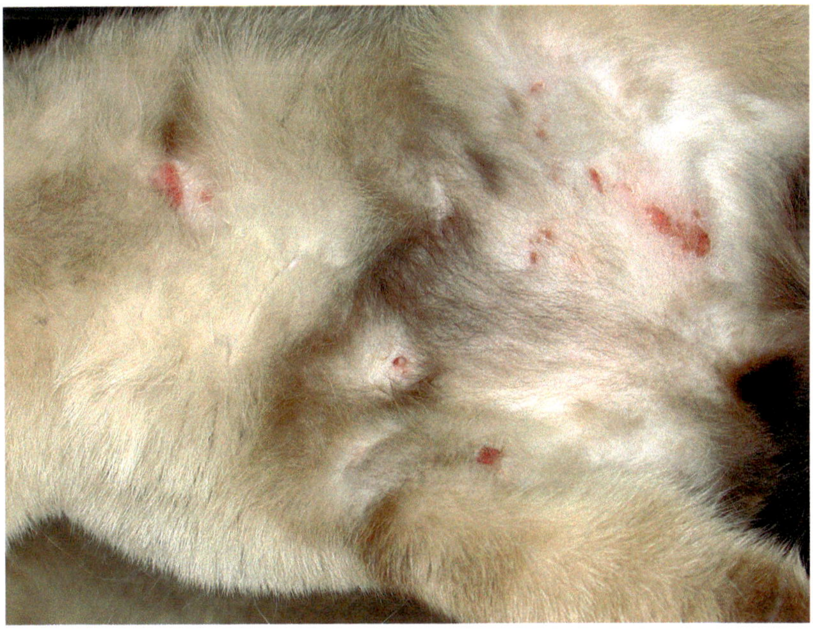

Figure 88.1. Appearance of the lesions in the inguinal area, with abscesses and chronic fistulous tracts.

Answers Case 88

1 What dermatological lesions does this cat have and what pathologies should be included in the differential diagnosis?

This cat's lesions are compatible with panniculitis of the inguinal subcutaneous fat. The differential diagnosis should include the following:

- Deep pyoderma with multiresistant bacteria.
- Nocardiosis.
- Actinomycosis.
- Mycobacteriosis.
- Subcutaneous mycosis.
- Nonseptic pyogranulomatous inflammatory processes (foreign bodies, sterile panniculitis).
- Neoplasms.

2 What diagnostic tests should be performed?

Ultrasound or computed tomography should be performed to rule out the presence of foreign bodies and determine the extent of the lesions. Other recommended tests include biopsy of the deep subcutaneous tissue for cytology and histology, culture, antibiogram, and in some cases molecular tests.

Case 89

Case presentation

An intact male mongrel dog, aged 14 years, was brought to the clinic by his owners with eczema that had appeared 2 months earlier. Despite treatment with cortisone and antibiotics, the lesions had not improved and had even progressively worsened. The dog appeared dejected, had lost weight, and licked his wounds. At the moment of the consultation, he was not receiving any treatment.

Apart from poor body condition, the results of the general examination were normal. In the dermatological examination, lesions were observed on the patient's ventral area (axillae, groin, skin of the abdomen) and on the inner aspect of the pinnae (Figs. 89.1–89.5).

Questions

1. What types of lesions are these?
2. What pathologies should be included in the differential diagnosis of this case?

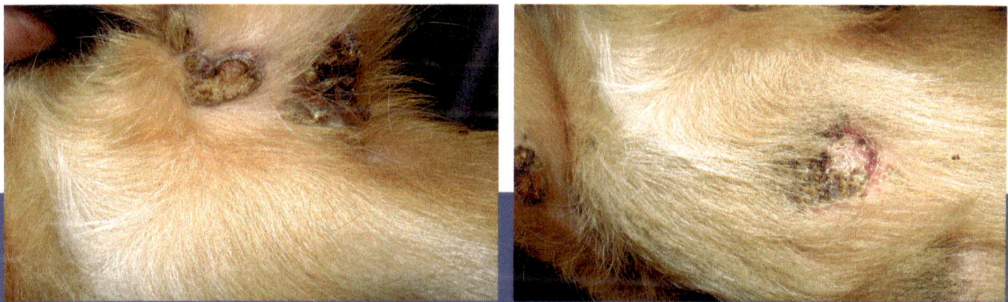

Figures 89.1 and 89.2. Skin lesions on the axillae and abdomen.

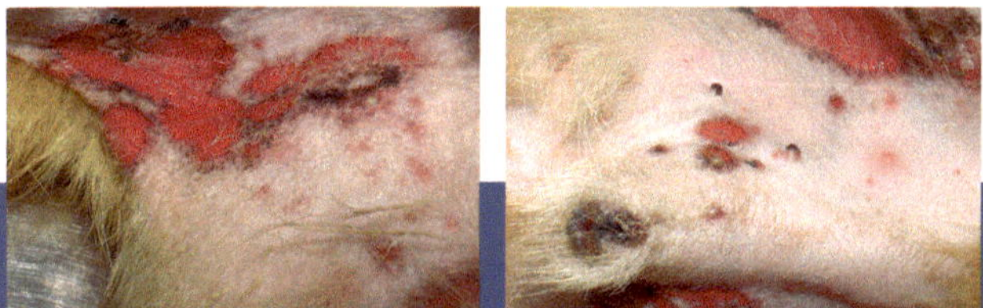

Figures 89.3 and 89.4. Appearance of the lesions after clipping and cleaning of the exudative and crusted tissue.

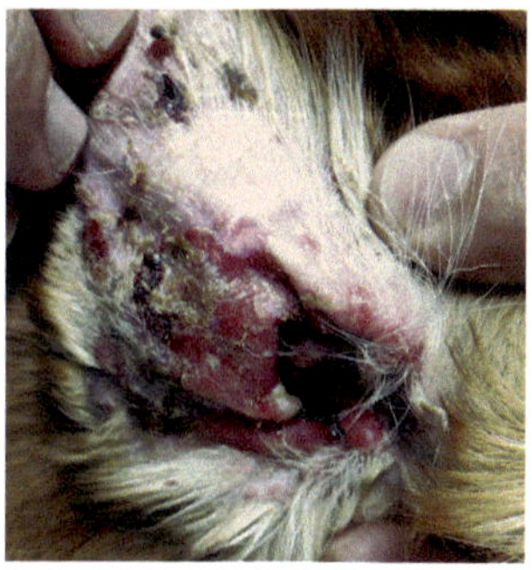

Figure 89.5. Appearance of the inner aspect of the pinna. ▶

Answers Case 89

1 What types of lesions are these?

These are highly exudative, crusted, and ulcerative multifocal lesions. Weight loss, depression, and ulcerative lesions are signs of a serious disease.

2 What pathologies should be included in the differential diagnosis of this case?

The differential diagnosis of ulcerative and crusted lesions in older animals should include the following:

- Primary neoplasms (epitheliotropic lymphoma, carcinoma *in situ*).
- Immune-mediated diseases (discoid or systemic lupus erythematosus, pemphigus vulgaris, erythema multiforme, toxic epidermal necrolysis, vasculitis).
- Infectious inflammatory causes (deep bacterial infections, atypical bacteria, deep mycoses, leishmaniasis).
- Nonseptic or traumatic inflammatory causes (thermal/chemical abrasions, solar dermatitis).

In this case, a skin biopsy revealed the presence of a multifocal squamous cell carcinoma *in situ* (Bowen's disease).

Observations

Bowen's disease is a multifocal neoplasia of keratinocytes. It can affect both pigmented and nonpigmented skin. It is a rare disease that mainly affects older dogs and has been associated with papillomavirus infections. The lesions are usually located around the mouth, in the genital area, and on the trunk. They can appear as pigmented plaques of 0.5 to 4 cm in diameter, which are usually alopecic, ulcerated, and painful, and can bleed significantly. These lesions tend to be chronic (lasting months to years) and can fluctuate in terms of severity (i.e. they improve and worsen, but do not disappear).

Diagnosis is established by histopathological examination, which reveals superficial epithelial dysplasia without involvement of the basement membrane. Hyperkeratosis and hypermelanosis are common and inflammatory exudate may be observed in cases of secondary infection. Hyperplasia and follicular dysplasias are also observed.

Case 90

Case presentation

A castrated male Persian cat, aged 1.5 years, presented with chronic facial pruritus that had appeared at 7 months of age. The cat had been placed on a hydrolysed diet for 8 weeks, with no improvement. He responded only to treatment with injectable corticosteroids, and for several months had received injections of methylprednisolone every 6 weeks, the only treatment that appeared to provide any relief. The last injection had been administered 4 weeks earlier. The cat had been purchased from a private breeder, had tested negative for feline leukaemia and immunodeficiency viruses, and lived all year round in an apartment. The owners administered fipronil by pipette once per month to control external parasites. The cat's general condition was good and apart from the facial pruritus, the animal was healthy. The owners of the cat had no skin lesions.

The results of the general examination were normal. In the dermatological examination mild erythema was observed on the eyelids and perioral area, as well as photophobia and the presence of a dark exudate with comedones around the eyelids and mouth and on the chin (Figs. 90.1–90.3). Some mild excoriation was also evident in the preauricular area. The examination revealed no other findings of note, and no lesions were observed in any other part of the body. Parasites were detected in the trichogram and in the scraping obtained from the lesions (Figs. 90.4 and 90.5).

Questions

1 What parasites are these?

2 Could they account for the patient's clinical signs?

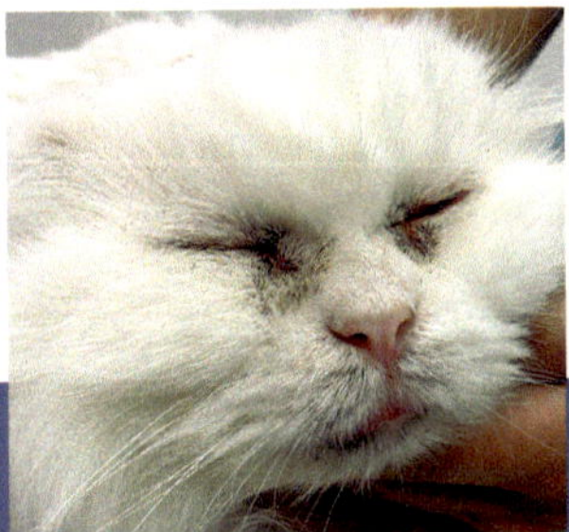

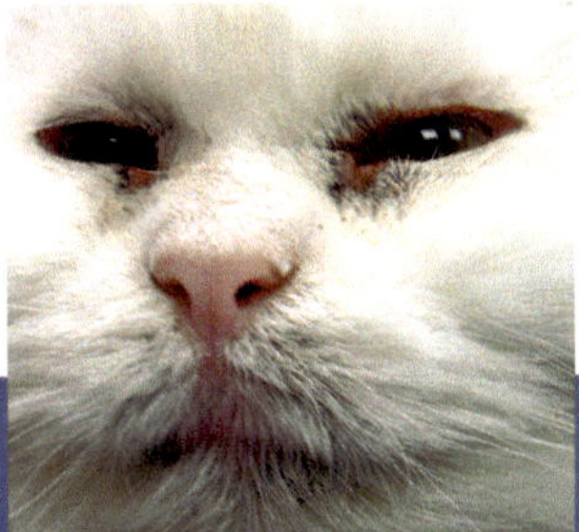

Figures 90.1 and 90.2. Photophobia, erythema of the eyelids, and dark exudate on the eyelids, lips, and chin.

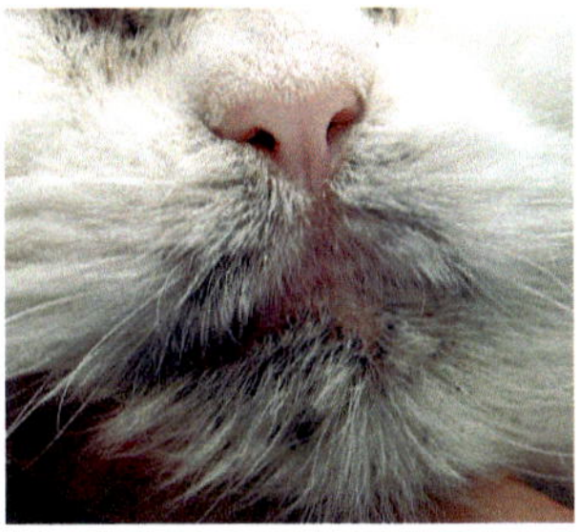

Figure 90.3. Detail showing dark exudate and comedones in the perioral area and chin.

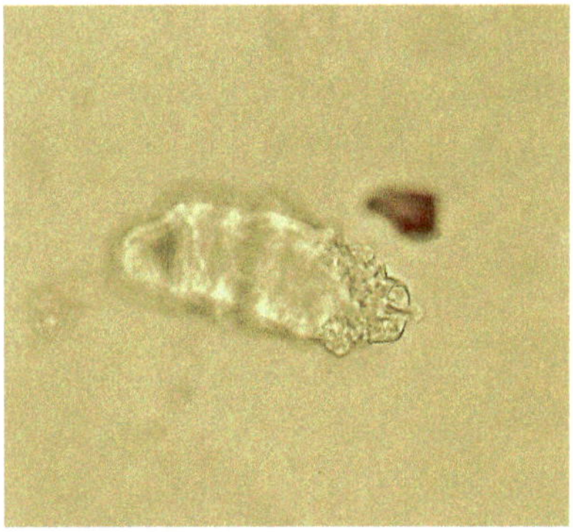

Figure 90.4. Mite.

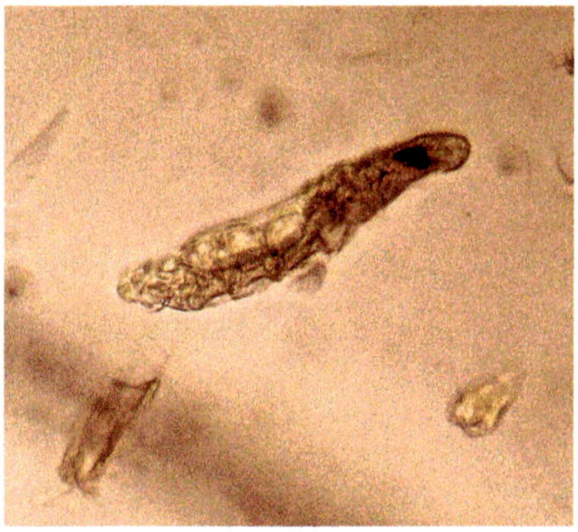

Figure 90.5. Mite.

Answers Case 90

1 What parasites are these?

Figures 90.4 and 90.5, respectively, show mites of the species *Demodex gatoi* and *Demodex cati*.

2 Could they account for the patient's clinical signs?

These two species of *Demodex* are parasites of cats. *D. gatoi* is contagious and can cause mild to moderate pruritus. *D. cati* infestations are more closely associated with systemic diseases that occur with immunosuppression, such as feline leukaemia virus infections, diabetes mellitus, hyperadrenocorticism, and neoplasms. In this clinical case, the presence of *D. cati* may have been due to the chronic administration of corticosteroids.

Treatments proposed for *D. gatoi* include calcium sulphide baths, ivermectin, milbemycin, and topical application (pipette) of moxidectin/imidacloprid. Because mites are sometimes difficult to observe in skin scrapings, therapeutic tests with acaricides may be indicated if this parasite is suspected. Infestation by *D. cati* is self-limiting, and resolves once the underlying cause is eliminated.

The patient was treated with calcium sulphide baths, which resulted in resolution of the exudative lesions and comedones. Skin scrapings obtained 4 weeks after starting treatment were negative. However, moderate facial pruritus persisted, and was controlled with oral cyclosporine administered twice per week.